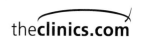

DENTAL CLINICS
OF NORTH AMERICA

Dental Public Health

GUEST EDITORS
Oscar Arevalo, DDS, ScD, MBA, MS and
Amit Chattopadhyay, PhD, MPH,
MDS, BDS (Hons)

April 2008 • Volume 52 • Number 2

SAUNDERS

An Imprint of Elsevier, Inc.
PHILADELPHIA LONDON TORONTO MONTREAL SYDNEY TOKYO

W.B. SAUNDERS COMPANY
A Division of Elsevier Inc.

Elsevier Inc. • 1600 John F. Kennedy Boulevard • Suite 1800 • Philadelphia, Pennsylvania 19103-2899

http://www.dental.theclinics.com

DENTAL CLINICS OF NORTH AMERICA Volume 52, Number 2
April 2008 ISSN 0011-8532
Editor: John Vassallo; j.vassallo@elsevier.com ISBN-13: 978-1-4160-5928-8
ISBN-10: 1-4160-5928-8

Dental Clinics of North America (ISSN 0011-8532) is published quarterly by Elsevier Inc., 360 Park Avenue South, New York, NY 10010-1710. Months of issue are January, April, July, and October. Business and Editorial Offices: 1600 John F. Kennedy Boulevard, Suite 1800, Philadelphia, PA 19103-2899. Customer Service Office: 6277 Sea Harbor Drive, Orlando, FL 32887-4800. Periodicals postage paid at New York, NY and additional mailing offices. Subscription prices are $188.00 per year (US individuals), $315.00 per year (US institutions), $91.00 per year (US students), $224.00 per year (Canadian individuals), $389.00 per year (Canadian institutions), $128.00 per year (Canadian students), $254.00 per year (international individuals), $389.00 per year (international institutions), and $128.00 per year (international students). International air speed delivery is included in all *Clinics* subscription prices. All prices are subject to change without notice. **POSTMASTER:** Send address changes to *Dental Clinics of North America*, Elsevier Periodicals Customer Service, 6277 Sea Harbor Drive, Orlando, FL 32887–4800. Customer Service: 1-800-654-2452 (US). From outside the United States, call 1-407-563-6020. Fax: 1-407-363-9661. E-mail: JournalsCustomerService-usa@elsevier.com.

The Dental Clinics of North America is covered in *Index Medicus, Current Contents/Clinical Medicine, ISI/BIOMED* and *Clinahl.*

Printed in the United States of America.

GUEST EDITORS

OSCAR AREVALO, DDS, ScD, MBA, MS, Assistant Professor and Chief, Division of Public Health, College of Dentistry, University of Kentucky, Lexington, Kentucky

AMIT CHATTOPADHYAY, PhD, MPH, MDS, BDS (Hons), Assistant Professor, Department of Epidemiology, University of Kentucky College of Public Health; and Assistant Professor, Division of Dental Public Health, Department of Oral Health Sciences, University of Kentucky College of Dentistry, Lexington, Kentucky

CONTRIBUTORS

OLUBUNMI ADEKUGBE, BDS, MPH, Dental Public Health Resident, New York State Department of Health, Albany, New York; Former Research Assistant, Massachusetts League of Community Health Centers, Boston, Massachusetts

MYRON ALLUKIAN, Jr, DDS, MPH, Oral Health Consultant, Massachusetts League of Community Health Centers; Lutheran Medical Center, Boston, Massachusetts

OSCAR AREVALO, DDS, ScD, MBA, MS, Assistant Professor and Chief, Division of Public Health, College of Dentistry, University of Kentucky, Lexington, Kentucky

HOWARD BAILIT, DMD, PhD, Professor Emeritus, Department of Community Medicine, School of Medicine, University of Connecticut, Farmington, Connecticut

TRYFON BEAZOGLOU, PhD, Professor, Department of Craniofacial Sciences, School of Dental Medicine, University of Connecticut, Farmington, Connecticut

CYNTHIA A. CADORET, RDH, MPH, Clinical Instructor, Department of Health Policy and Health Services Research; and Co-Investigator, Northeast Center for Research to Evaluate and Eliminate Dental Disparities, Boston University Goldman School of Dental Medicine, Boston, Massachusetts

J.M. CHALMERS, BDSc, MS, PhD, Associate Professor, Department of Preventive and Community Dentistry, College of Dentistry, The University of Iowa, Iowa City, Iowa

AMIT CHATTOPADHYAY, PhD, MPH, MDS, BDS (Hons), Assistant Professor, Department of Epidemiology, University of Kentucky College of Public Health; and Assistant Professor, Division of Dental Public Health, Department of Oral Health Sciences, University of Kentucky College of Dentistry, Lexington, Kentucky

R.L. ETTINGER, BDS, MDS, DDSc, Professor, Department of Preventive and Community Dentistry, College of Dentistry, The University of Iowa, Iowa City, Iowa

RAUL I. GARCIA, DMD, MMedSc, Professor and Chair, Department of Health Policy and Health Services Research; and Director, Northeast Center for Research to Evaluate and Eliminate Dental Disparities, Boston University Goldman School of Dental Medicine, Boston, Massachusetts

PAUL GLASSMAN, DDS, MA, MBA, Professor of Dental Practice, and Associate Dean for Information and Educational Technology, and Director of the Advanced Education in General Dentistry Program, University of the Pacific, Arthur A. Dugoni School of Dentistry, San Francisco, California

MICHELLE HENSHAW, DDS, MPH, Associate Professor, Department of Health Policy and Health Services Research; and Co-Director, Northeast Center for Research to Evaluate and Eliminate Dental Disparities; and Assistant Dean, Community Partnership and Extramural Affairs, Boston University Goldman School of Dental Medicine, Boston, Massachusetts

ALICE M. HOROWITZ, PhD, Advisor to the Dean on Health Literacy, Office of the Dean, School of Public Health, University of Maryland, College Park, Maryland

DUSHANKA V. KLEINMAN, DDS, MScD, Associate Dean for Research, School of Public Health, University of Maryland, College Park, Maryland

JAYANTH V. KUMAR, DDS, MPH, Director, Oral Health Surveillance and Research, Bureau of Dental Health, New York State Department of Health; Associate Professor, School of Public Health, University at Albany, Albany, New York

MARK E. MOSS, DDS, MS, PhD, Consultant Public Health Dentist, Bureau of Dental Health, New York State Department of Health; Private Practitioner, InterLakes Health, Ticonderoga, New York

BHAVNA T. PAHEL, BDS, MPH, Department of Health Policy and Administration, School of Public Health, University of North Carolina at Chapel Hill, Chapel Hill, North Carolina

R. GARY ROZIER, DDS, MPH, Department of Health Policy and Administration, School of Public Health, University of North Carolina at Chapel Hill, Chapel Hill, North Carolina

WOOSUNG SOHN, DDS, MS, PhD, DrPH, Assistant Professor, Department of Cariology, Restorative Sciences and Endodontics, Health Services and Epidemiology Research Unit, University of Michigan School of Dentistry; Adjunct Assistant Professor, Department of Epidemiology, University of Michigan School of Public Health, Ann Arbor, Michigan

PAUL SUBAR, DDS, Assistant Professor of Dental Practice, University of the Pacific, Arthur A. Dugoni School of Dentistry, San Francisco, California

SCOTT L. TOMAR, DMD, DrPH, Professor and Chair, Department of Community Dentistry and Behavioral Science, University of Florida College of Dentistry, Gainesville, Florida

CONTENTS

Dental public health is a unique and challenging American Dental Association-recognized specialty because the patient is the entire community or population, such as a school, neighborhood, city, state, or the nation, with a focus on vulnerable populations. Limited resources are maximized through prevention, policies, programs, and organized community efforts to respond to great unmet needs. Although dental public health professionals are few in number, millions of people every day have better oral health because of these professionals, who work on the local, state, and national level.

This article examines the financing of dental care in the United States. The major issues addressed include the amount and sources of funds, the reasons for increased dental care expenditures, the comparison of dental care with other medical care expenditures, the policy implications of current trends, and some cautious predictions about the financing of dental care in the next 10 to 20 years. The supply of dental services is expected to increase substantially in the next 10 to 20 years with more dental school graduates, a new midlevel practitioner, and greater use of allied dental health personnel. Whether the supply of services will grow faster than the demand for care is unknown.

from the perspective of oral health-related quality of life (OHRQoL), yet available evidence shows that a substantial percentage of the adult population rates their oral health poorly. This article reviews applications of OHRQoL in dental public health. The authors specifically review its use, contributions, and needed advances in: (1) monitoring the impacts of oral diseases on OHRQoL at the national level, and in public health surveillance at the state and local levels, (2) treatment outcomes research and program evaluation; and (3) clinical practice.

A general understanding of the measurement of dental diseases can help practitioners in the process of assessing the patient's future risk of disease. More importantly, as clinical studies shift from the traditional academic setting to practice-based networks, practitioners might play a more significant role in research. An important issue in oral health disease management in the future will be the standardization of clinical criteria and the development of alternative mechanisms of data collection for epidemiologic purposes.

The use of fluorides in dental public health programs has a long history. With the availability of fluoridation and other forms of fluorides, dental caries have declined dramatically in the United States. This article reviews some of the ways fluorides are used in public health programs and discusses issues related to their effectiveness, cost, and policy.

Community oral-health programs focus primarily on populations, including those who do not seek oral health care. Planning these programs should include involvement of the community, broadly defined to include individuals and organizations that represent those who can help design and implement it and those who could be affected by it. This article provides an overview of systematic approaches to planning and evaluating community oral health programs. Such approaches help ensure that stakeholders agree on the purpose of the program, work toward its success, and contribute toward its continuous improvement.

The aging United States population living in the new millennium has dental needs that are very different and more complex than those experienced by previous older adult cohorts during the twentieth century. The type of dental care to be provided for older Americans goes way beyond emergency care, extractions and denture care. Dental caries is still clearly a public health problem for subgroups of older Americans, such as those of lower socioeconomic status, with dementia, who are homebound and who are institutionalized. These are also the subgroups experiencing greater barriers to accessing dental care. Stakeholders, including dental professionals and the dental benefits industry, need to work together to develop innovative dental financing programs that will increase older Americans access to dental care.

The number of people in the United States population with disabilities and other special needs is growing dramatically. These individuals present unique challenges for oral health professionals in planning and carrying out dental treatment and for the oral health delivery system. Because it has been recognized that the current delivery system is not working well for these populations, new workforce, financing, and delivery models are beginning to emerge that may hold promise for creating and maintaining oral health for currently underserved populations, including people with disabilities and other special needs. This article discusses the implications of this for the oral health profession, describes the challenges of providing oral health services for this population, and discusses the implications of these challenges for the organization of the oral health delivery system.

FORTHCOMING ISSUES

RECENT ISSUES

ELSEVIER
SAUNDERS

Dent Clin N Am 52 (2008) xi–xii

THE DENTAL
CLINICS
OF NORTH AMERICA

Preface

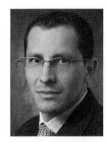 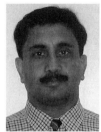

Oscar Arevalo, DDS, ScD,   Amit Chattopadhyay, PhD, MPH,
MBA, MS   MDS, BDS (Hons)
Guest Editors

This issue of *Dental Clinics of North America* is a succinct examination of the discipline of dental public health. As guest editors, we have provided a platform on which the many facets of the discipline could be presented and describe its vast domain and truly interdisciplinary nature. We expect that the readers of this issue will develop a deeper understanding of the relevance of dental public health to the practice of clinical dentistry. In the interest of brevity and trimming redundancy, topics related to dental public health that have been addressed by other recent issues of *Dental Clinics of North America* were not included here.

While this publication is in production, the presidential primaries are underway. Once again, access to health care and the increasing expenditures for health care services are being debated intensely. Changes in the organization and financing of health care leading to an increased number of individuals covered by social insurance programs could have positive consequences for the oral health status of Americans. Reports at the state and national levels are focusing on access to dental care, particularly for underserved populations. In addition, many other converging factors will present enormous challenges to the dental care delivery system over the next decade, including an aging population, changes in the ethnic composition of the country, dental student debt levels, minority and special needs populations' health disparities, limited health care dollars for oral health, and ineffective delivery systems.

As solutions to these challenges are explored, the role of the discipline of dental public health seems destined to expand its responsibility and sphere of influence. As a clinical specialist, the public health dentist provides direct care in public health settings. In addition, he or she participates in the planning, implementation, and evaluation of preventive and therapeutic programs, placing substantial emphasis on populations that have difficulties accessing the dental care delivery system. Although the role of public health dentists is important, the development and implementation of large systemic solutions will require the input, active involvement, and expertise of professional associations, dental educators, researchers, public health agencies, private industry, and consumer groups. In this issue, the contributing authors have pointed this out from their different perspectives.

Any publication is a collaborative enterprise. Certainly, a publication such as this one, where the work of various contributors is integrated, owes much to the work of many individuals. As editors, we were responsible for the selection of topics and contributors, and we provided feedback to authors for improvements in their articles. This publication has benefited from the inspiration, cooperation, and wisdom of many people: notably, Dr. Richard Haug at the University of Kentucky College of Dentistry for championing this idea, and Mr. John Vassallo at Elsevier/Saunders for his substantial support and ample guidance in putting this issue together. Most of all, this publication owes its content to a committed group of experts who readily agreed to contribute to this issue despite their busy schedules.

Oral health is an integral component of general health and well-being and a basic human right. As such, it must be available and attainable by all Americans.

Oscar Arevalo, DDS, ScD, MBA, MS
Division of Dental Public Health
College of Dentistry
University of Kentucky
Suite 101
333 Waller Avenue
Lexington, KY 40504, USA

E-mail address: oarev2@email.uky.edu

Amit Chattopadhyay, PhD, MPH, MDS, BDS (Hons)
Department of Epidemiology
University of Kentucky
College of Public Health
Room # 209-C
121 Washington Avenue
Lexington, KY 40536, USA

E-mail address: achat4@email.uky.edu

ELSEVIER
SAUNDERS

THE DENTAL
CLINICS
OF NORTH AMERICA

Dent Clin N Am 52 (2008) 259–280

The Practice and Infrastructure of Dental Public Health in the United States

Myron Allukian, Jr, DDS, MPH[a,b,*],
Olubunmi Adekugbe, BDS, MPH[a,c]

[a]Massachusetts League of Community Health Centers, 40 Court Street,
10th Floor, Boston, MA 02108, USA
[b]Lutheran Medical Center, 40 Court Street, 10th Floor, Boston, MA 02108, USA
[c]New York State Department of Health,
Room 532 ESP Corning Tower, Albany, NY 12237, USA

A 45-year-old man who has AIDS has been robbed and is in pain with a number of broken teeth. He calls at least 25 dentists in his community for treatment… they all refuse to treat him.

A state with a population of 6 million people is only 8% fluoridated, and the public must vote before the Board of Health can order fluoridation. The average 16-year-old in the state has 15 teeth affected by tooth decay.

A state's governor eliminates the adult dental Medicaid program because it's "too expensive."

A 10-year-old boy who has a throbbing abscess is terrified to go to the dentist and wants all his teeth removed with "gas."

A mother of a developmentally disabled child cannot find a dentist anywhere near her home to treat her child.

Dental care is the most requested health service of a state Medicaid program, with 4,000 calls a month, followed by mental health, with 700.

A school nurse is frustrated by the number of children who need dental care but cannot afford it.

A city mayor wants to develop a citywide program to improve the quality of life for the homeless population.

A nonfluoridated community, where 24% of the children of the low-income children screened have dental pain and infection, wants to become fluoridated.

An inner city neighborhood wants to know whether dentistry should be included in their newly developing community health center.

* Corresponding author. 46 Louders Lane, Boston, MA 02130.
  E-mail address: myalluk@aol.com (M. Allukian, Jr).

0011-8532/08/$ - see front matter © 2008 Elsevier Inc. All rights reserved.
doi:10.1016/j.cden.2007.12.003

dental.theclinics.com

These are examples of public health problems and underserved populations who need the expertise and assistance of dental public health professionals. Dental public health professionals make a significant difference in the quality of life of millions of people in the communities they serve throughout the United States each year.

Dental public health professionals are responsible for the oral health of a population or a group of individuals, in contrast to the dental clinician or private practitioner who is primarily responsible for the oral health of the individual patient sophisticated enough to seek them out and who has resources to pay for services. The dental public health professional may work for a community, city, county, state, or federal government, or in an academic or research setting, or for an institution, organization, agency, or company involved in oral health or oral health products.

The unique expertise of the dental public professional is essential for dealing with population groups in terms of administration, policy, programs, prevention, and research. The dental public health infrastructure has as its major responsibility to promote, protect, and enhance the oral health of the community or population they serve. This population may be schools, neighborhoods, nursing homes, towns, cities, states, or the nation, or a combination of these different communities. Not only does the dental public health professional help the whole community, but he or she also focuses on vulnerable or high-risk populations, such as children, the elderly, the low income, the developmentally disabled, the medically comprised, the homebound or homeless, persons with HIV/AIDS, uninsured and institutionalized individuals, and racial, cultural, and linguistic minorities [1].

Dental public health: definition, scope, and practice

The American Association of Public Health Dentistry defines dental public health as "....the science and art of preventing and controlling dental diseases and promoting dental health through organized community efforts. It is that form of dental practice which serves the community as a patient rather than the individual. It is concerned with the dental education of the public, with applied dental research, and with the administration of group dental care programs as well as the prevention and control of dental diseases on a community basis" [2].

Dental public health is probably the most challenging specialty of dentistry because almost everyone has the disease, most people periodically have new disease, the patient is the entire population or community, the resources are limited, and the impact is enormous.

Specialty recognition

Dental public health was established as a specialty in 1950, and is one of the nine specialties of dentistry currently recognized by the American Dental

Association (ADA). In 1986, it was the first of the then eight specialties of dentistry to be reviewed and receive continued recognition as a specialty, and then was reviewed again in 1996. It is the only specialty that deals with population groups and is the second smallest in number of active board certified specialists, having only 155 active diplomates in 2006 [3]. To become board certified a dentist must have a master's degree in public health and have completed a dental public health residency or its educational equivalent, have 2 years of public health experience, and must pass the examination of the American Board of Dental Public Health.

In 2007, there were 38 accredited schools of public health and 13 dental public health residency training programs in the United States. There are approximately 2,032 dentists in the United States who work in public health and about 1,000 of these have at least 1 year of advanced education beyond dental school; over 600 have 2 years of advanced education beyond dental school [4]. Dental hygiene does not have recognized specialization of any kind; however, some public health dental hygienists have advanced degrees in public health.

Scope and practice of dental public health

Dental public health expertise is needed wherever one is concerned about oral health and groups of people, or populations of concern. Education and training in such areas as epidemiology, biostatistics, policy, management, administration, and research, give the public health professional the tools to help a population achieve better oral health.

Core competencies: there are certain core competencies a dental public health professional must have to be effective in the practice of public health. In 1988, the 165 competency objectives covered the following four broad categories:

- Health policy and program management
- Research methods in dental public health
- Oral health promotion and disease prevention
- Oral health services and delivery

In 1997, the dental public health leadership narrowed these objectives to 10 competencies with an emphasis on skills, not just knowledge, as in earlier editions. The specialist trained in dental public health is expected to have skills in these 10 core competencies (Box 1) [5].

This list includes competencies necessary for planning (I), implementing, monitoring, and evaluating oral health programs (V, VI) at the community level (III, VII). The interventions to control oral health disease and promote oral health (II) are based on needs (VI, IX, X). The competency requirements mandate that interventions should be based on scientifically proven, cost effective, and ethical standards (IV, II, IX). Other competency requirements include advocacy for oral health policy (VIII), sound management skills (III), and the ability to interpret and translate science to recommendations for

---

Box 1. Ten dental public health competencies (AAPHD)

   I. Plan oral health programs for populations.
  II. Select interventions and strategies for the prevention
      and control of oral diseases and promotion of oral health
 III. Develop resources, implement and manage oral health
      programs for populations
  IV. Incorporate ethical standards in oral health programs and
      activities
   V. Evaluate and monitor dental care delivery systems
  VI. Design and understand the use of surveillance systems
      to monitor oral health
 VII. Communicate and collaborate with groups and individuals on
      oral health issues
VIII. Advocate for, implement, and evaluate public health policy,
      legislation, and regulations to protect and promote the
      public's oral health
  IX. Critique and synthesize scientific literature
   X. Design and conduct population-based studies to answer oral
      and public health questions

Adapted from Preamble to the Competency Statements for Dental Public
Health. J Public Health Dent 1998;58(S1):119–20; with permission. Available at:
http://www.aaphd.org/default.asp?page=competencies.htm. Accessed August 20,
2007.

---

action (IX). Other basic skills needed by dental public health professionals
include knowledge of clinical dentistry, leadership, and communication skills,
and the ability to work effectively with coalitions and constituency building.
Thus, being a competent and effective dental public health professional
requires many skills and competencies to be successful.

Dental workforce education, licensure, and regulation

One of the roles of the dental public health specialist is to determine and
influence how the dental workforce may better serve the public. The total
number of dentists in the United States in 2004 was 175,705, with 92.3%
in private practice. There are about 60 dentists per 100,000 people [6,7]. The
closure of seven dental schools in earlier years and the increasing cost of dental
education have led to a decrease in the number of graduates. The ratio of
dentists to people is expected to drop to 52.7 per 100,000 by the year 2020 [8].

There are approximately 54 dental hygienists per 100,000 people nationally, with a total of 158,269 hygienists in 2005. There are about 91 dental
hygienists for every 100 dentists nationally. The total number of dental

assistants was 268,940 in 2005. The ratio of dental assistants to dentists was 1.54 and the number of dental assistants per 100,000 people was 91.58 [6].

In the United States, as of 2004, there were 56 dental schools and 266 and 259 dental hygiene and dental assisting programs, respectively [9]. The number of dental graduates increased by 18% from 1992–1993 to 2003–2004, while the number of dental hygiene graduates increased by over 50% from 1992–1993 to 2003–2004 [10].

The practice of dentistry and dental hygiene is regulated by the laws of individual states as per the State Dental Practice Act. All states and the District of Columbia have a Board of Dentistry, a Board of Dental Examiners, or a state Dental Commission, which enforce the state dental laws and develop rules and regulations based on the laws. These boards may affect the scope of practice of the dentist, dental hygienist, and dental assistant, and have a significant impact on the public's oral health and the practice of dental public health. Immediate consequences of these variations are differences in the amount of supervision under which a dental hygienist can practice and the scope of service hygienists and dental assistants may provide. Hygienists can ease access to oral health services and prevention programs for the underserved, especially in public health programs. In 2002, only one state allowed a dental hygienist to perform a prophylaxis without any form of supervision [10]. In 2007, 22 states allowed direct access to a hygienist, 12 states allowed them to bill Medicaid, and 45 states allowed dental hygienists to practice under general supervision [11].

Dental public health infrastructure

The infrastructure for dental public health is the foundation upon which public dental programs and activities are assessed, planned, executed, and evaluated. Unfortunately, this workforce and infrastructure is under-appreciated and a low priority of our society in general, with limited resources to meet the great unmet oral health needs of our country. The Surgeon General's Report on Oral Health noted that "the public health infrastructure for oral health is insufficient to address the needs of disadvantaged groups, and the integration of oral and general health programs is lacking" [12].

The different levels of government—federal, state, and local or county— have the potential to make a significant impact on a community's oral health. Many public health dentists and dental hygienists work for federal, state, or local government. These agencies and infrastructure impact the lives of millions of people and are described in the following sections.

The US Department of Health and Human Services, the federal dental public health infrastructure and programs

The US Department of Health and Human Services (HHS) is the principal federal agency that administers public health programs in the United

States. The HHS has a stated priority of protecting the health of all Americans and providing essential human services, especially for those least able to help themselves. The President's budget for the HHS for fiscal year (FY) 2008 was $698 billion, and the HHS has approximately 66,890 full-time equivalent employees (FTEs) of personnel [13].

Dentistry's recent history in the HHS

In the 1960s and 1970s dentistry had a significant role in the HHS, with over 300 personnel in the Division of Dentistry, and public health dentists in all ten public health service regional offices. This was the heyday of public health activity through the federal sector, with the development of many new public health programs such as Medicare, Medicaid, Head Start, Community and Migrant Health Centers, Community Action Programs, and the National Health Service Corps, to name a few, all with significant dental components, except Medicare. In the late 1970s and 1980s, there was a major decline in dentistry's role in the HHS, as the Division of Dentistry decreased to a handful of personnel. The National Health Service Corps dental field strength dropped from 500 in 1982 to 50 in 1989, fluoridation activities were moved to the then Centers for Disease Control, the dental public health residency training grants were not reauthorized, and the support for training dental auxillaries and personnel in team practice was also discontinued in 1981, while support for training physician assistants and nurse practitioners continued. The 1989 Final Report to Congress on Oral Health Activities documented the diminished role of dentistry in the HHS [14,15].

After much activity by the dental public health community, in the 1990s oral health was included in the White House's national health plan, the Secretary of the HHS began an Oral Health Initiative, and dental public health residencies were reauthorized by Congress. In 1992, a Chief Dental Officer was selected for the Health Resources and Services Administration (HRSA) and oral health was made a priority in this agency again. The Secretary's Oral Health Initiative included workforce development, direct service, improving the dental public health infrastructure, and translating science into practice and policy. The Surgeon General's Report on Oral Health, which was several years in the making, was released in 2000. In 2000, with the new administration, the HRSA Chief Dental Officer position was abolished, but reinstituted in 2007.

During the 1980s and 1990s, it was also very helpful to the public's oral health that oral health was included in the 1990 National Health Objectives, as well as Healthy People 2000 and Healthy People 2010. Also beginning in the early 1970s, the then National Institute of Dental Research (NIDR), now the National Institute of Dental and Craniofacial Research (NIDCR), played a very significant role in community based prevention initiatives, such as community water fluoridation, school fluoridation, school fluoride programs, and pit and fissure sealants. NIDR also demonstrated that school-based plaque control programs did not prevent caries, but did help prevent gingivitis. In the 1990s, the funding of the Centers for Research to Reduce Oral Health Disparities was initiated.

The oral health activities undertaken by two federal offices and specific federal agencies are described in the following sections.

Office of the Surgeon General

The Surgeon General is the nation's chief health educator, appointed by the President and confirmed by the Senate, and reports to the Secretary of Health and Human Services. In 2000, the first ever Surgeon General's Report on Oral Health described the magnitude of oral diseases in the United States population and the actions necessary to address them [12]. The Report is available at www.surgeongeneral.gov/library/oralhealth. Major findings of the report were:

- Oral diseases and disorders in and of themselves affect health and well being throughout life.
- Safe and effective measures exist to prevent the most common dental diseases—dental caries and periodontal diseases.
- Lifestyle behaviors that affect general health, such as tobacco use, excessive alcohol use, and poor dietary choices affect oral and craniofacial health as well.
- There are profound and consequential oral health disparities within the United States population.
- More information is needed to improve America's oral health and eliminate health disparities.
- The mouth reflects general health and well being.
- Oral diseases and conditions are associated with other health problems.
- Scientific research is key to further reduction in the burden of diseases and disorders that affect the face, mouth, and teeth.

The Surgeon General's Report on Oral Health and the National Call to Action to Promote Oral Health had a significant impact on raising the visibility of the silent epidemic of oral diseases. The Call to Action is available at http://www.surgeongeneral.gov/topics/oralhealth/nationalcalltoaction.htm.

Office of Disease Prevention and Health Promotion
and Healthy People 2010

Healthy People 2010 is a set of health objectives for the nation to be achieved over the first decade of this century and administered by the Office of Disease Prevention and Health Promotion. Oral health is one of 28 priority areas, with 17 objectives and many subobjectives. The oral health objectives are for preventing and controlling oral and craniofacial diseases, conditions, and injuries, and improving access to related services [16]. Goals 21 to 14 and 21 to 17 are related to increasing the proportion of oral health programs and dental public health personnel in federal, state, and local agencies. Healthy People 2010 is available at www.healthypeople.gov.

The United States Public Health Service

The United States Public Health Service Commissioned Corps is a uniformed service of more than 6,000 health professionals who serve in the HHS and other federal agencies. The Surgeon General heads this uniformed commissioned corps. The Chief Dental Officer is appointed by the United States Surgeon General and is responsible for providing leadership, coordination, and professional growth of the dental personnel in the Public Health Service (PHS).

In 2007, there were 389 dental officers in the PHS Commissioned Corps, which constituted 8.2% of all Commissioned Corps officers [15]. In 2004, 51% of the Commissioned Corps dental officers were assigned to the Indian Health Service (IHS), 23% to the Bureau of Prisons, and 11% to the Department of Homeland Security. The 114 institutions under the Bureau of Prisons are responsible for the care of almost 200,000 inmates [17].

Indian Health Service

The IHS is the primary health care provider and health care advocate for American Indian and Alaska Native communities. The IHS employs approximately 15,550 people from a variety of professional backgrounds, with an expenditure of $2.2 billion in 2005 to serve a population of 2.5 million eligible Native Americans dispersed across 35 states in 557 different federally recognized tribes [18]. The IHS has been actively involved in the development of programs to address the oral health needs of rural Alaska Natives who have great difficulty in accessing oral health services [19].

In FY 2006, the Division of Oral Health had a budget of $117.7 million and there were 489 full-time dentists and 147 full-time dental hygienists in the field [20]. There are currently 148 dentist vacancies at the IHS, a vacancy rate of 33%, which is higher than for any other profession [21].

Centers for Disease Control and Prevention

The mission of Centers for Disease Control and Prevention (CDC) is to promote health and quality of life by preventing and controlling disease, injury, and disability. The President's budget for the CDC for FY 2008 was $8.8 billion [22]. The Division of Oral Health (DOH) is one of ten Divisions within the National Center for Chronic Disease Prevention and Health Promotion. There are ten dental public health personnel in the DOH. Its strategic priorities are:

- Strengthening the capacity of state oral health programs
- Improving the capacity to monitor the nation's oral health
- Building the evidence base to strengthen prevention strategies
- Disseminating data, findings, and effective prevention practices [23]

The budget for the DOH has increased from $3 million in FY 1998 to $11.6 million in FY 2007. The DOH helps states, territories, and other countries collect oral health data, apply new methods for oral health surveillance, monitor the status of community water fluoridation, and train state and local fluoridation engineers and state program leaders on fluoridation. The DOH also promotes and provides technical assistance on school-based and school-linked dental sealant programs, investigates outbreaks of infectious diseases in clinical dental settings, and provides infection control information for dental personnel and serves as a resource within CDC on oral health [24].

National Center for Health Statistics

The National Center for Health Statistics (NCHS) is the nation's principal agency for providing health statistics and it is a part of the CDC. This information is used to develop policies and programs to improve health. Oral health-related activities at the NCHS are primarily concentrated in the Division of Health and Nutrition Examination Surveys, which is responsible for planning, implementing, conducting, and evaluating examination and nutrition surveys at NCHS.

National Institutes of Health

The National Institutes of Health (NIH) is the primary federal agency conducting and supporting medical research, with an annual budget of over $28 billion [25]. The discoveries from these institutes have prevented diseases and improved the quality of people's lives. This 100-year HHS agency achieves this by awarding competitive grants to researchers in its own laboratories, universities, medical and dental schools, and other research institutions. The NIH is made up of 27 different components, called institutes and centers, with specific research agendas, such as the National Cancer Institute, National Institute of Mental Health, and others.

National Institute of Dental and Craniofacial Research is one of the NIH Institutes. The organizational mission is accomplished by:

- Performing and supporting basic and clinical research
- Conducting and funding research training and career development programs to ensure an adequate number of talented, well-prepared, and diverse investigators
- Coordinating and assisting relevant research and research-related activities among all sectors of the research community
- Promoting the timely transfer of knowledge gained from research and implications for health to the public, health professionals, researchers, and policy-makers [24].

The NIDCR Division of Extramural Research plans, develops, and manages basic, translational, and clinical research supported by grants, cooperative agreements, and contracts in dental, oral, and craniofacial health and disease. Some of the areas into which research is being done include infectious diseases, health disparities, behavioral and social aspects of health and disease, temporomandibular joint dysfunction, developmental biology and mammalian genetics, AIDS and oral manifestations of immunosuppression, biomaterials, and tissue engineering and regenerative medicine [25]. The NIDCR's FY 2007 budget was $389.4 million [26].

Centers for Medicare and Medicaid Services

The Centers for Medicare and Medicaid Services (CMS) is the federal agency responsible for administering the Medicare, Medicaid, State Children's Health Insurance (SCHIP), the Health Insurance Portability and Accountability Act, the Clinical Laboratory Improvement Amendments, and several other health-related programs. The total CMS expenditure (Medicaid, SCHIP, and Medicare) on all health services was $660 billion and spending for dental services was only $4.9 billion [27]. National expenditures for dental care were over $86.6 billion in 2005, or 4.4% of total health care expenditures, a continuing decrease from 6.4% in 1970 [28]. The percentage of the population without health insurance has been on the increase; in 2006 it was 15.8%, or about 47 million people, with the majority being ethnic minorities [29]. In 2004, 34.6% of all Americans had no dental coverage, more than twice the number without medical insurance [30].

The dental public health workforce is often intimately involved on the national, state, and local level, helping to improve these CMS programs and to provide access to these resources for vulnerable populations. There are two public health dentists who work in the CMS.

Medicare is the federal government sponsored and funded health insurance program that covers people who are older than 65 years and people less than 65 years who have certain disabilities or end-stage renal disease. It is administered in Parts A, B, C, and D or hospital care, outpatient visits, and prescription drugs. About 41 million Americans are covered under Medicare at a cost of about $342 billion in 2005 [31]. Dental benefits are not routinely covered under Medicare, except under certain conditions, such as oral cancer [32]. In 2005 the Medicare expenditure for dental services was $92 million [27].

Medicaid is the federal and state funded program that offers care to eligible low-income individuals and families. As of 2004, about 58.5 million Americans were covered under Medicaid, with about 50% being children, at a total cost of about $310 billion, of which 57% is federal money and 43% state money. Many more are eligible for these programs, however they are not enrolled. The expenditure for dental services from Medicaid for 2005 was $4.2 billion, or 1.35% [27]. Dental care is mandatory for children and optional for adults, being determined by the states. In most states, access to dental care is inadequate for children on Medicaid, with only 15.7% actually receiving treatment in 2004, primarily because dentists do not participate in the program [32–34].

State Child Health Insurance Program

SCHIP is jointly financed by the federal and state governments. In some states the program is a part of the state Medicaid program. The states are allowed flexibility within federal guidelines on the benefits covered. SCHIP builds on Medicaid coverage and provides additional access for up to 6 million low-income children. Dental benefits are covered by all states but one [34]. However, given the amount of discretion allowed at the state level on benefits, it is not uncommon to have cuts in dental benefits. Total Medicaid SCHIP expansion and SCHIP expenses for 2005 was $7.6 billion, with dental expenses making up 7.3% or $563 million of the total [27].

Food and Drug Administration

The Food and Drug Administration (FDA) is responsible for protecting the public's health by assuring the safety, efficacy, and security of human and veterinary drugs, biologic products, medical devices, our nation's food supply, cosmetics, and products that emit radiation. The FDA currently employs five dental professionals.

Health Resources and Services Administration

The primary purpose of the Health Resources and Services Administration is to improve access to health care services for people who are uninsured, isolated, or medically vulnerable [35]. HRSA grantees provide health care in all states to uninsured people, people living with HIV/AIDS, and pregnant women, mothers, and children. HRSA activities are managed centrally and through the ten public health service regions, some of which have dental consultants with mostly nondental responsibilities. The bureaus most active in oral health are HIV/AIDS, Maternal and Child Health, Primary Health Care, and Health Professions.

The HIV/AIDS Bureau provides clinical care and support for uninsured and underinsured individuals and families of individuals with HIV/AIDS. Through the Ryan White Care Act in FY 2006, 78,000 clients with 220,000 encounters received oral health services at a cost of $43 million in the Parts A, B, C, and D programs (HIV Bureau, Health Resources and Services Administration Department of Health and Human Services, personal communication, 2007).

The Maternal and Child Health Bureau (MCHB) is responsible for assuring that necessary services are made available to American mothers and children. Programs coordinated by the MCHB, which include oral health, have as their objective to support the development and implementation of comprehensive, culturally competent, coordinated systems of care for the estimated 18 million United States children who have or are at risk for chronic, physical, developmental, behavioral, or emotional conditions, and who also require health and related services of a type or amount beyond that required by children generally [36]. Expenditures by the federal government on maternal and child health services were $628 million in 2005 [27]. Dental expenditures were 2.1% or about $13 million.

Other efforts of the MCHB include the National Oral Health Policy Center, which provides information and support for national, state, and local (MCHB) programs; develops policy that advances oral health and dental care for (MCHB) populations and vulnerable and at-risk populations; and supports leadership development in oral health policy [37].

The National Maternal and Child Oral Health Resource Center aims to support health professionals, program administrators, educators, policy-makers, and others with the goal of improving oral health services for pregnant women, infants, children, and adolescents, including those with special health care needs and their families [38]. Activities of the Oral Health Resource Center include collecting programmatic materials, such as guidelines, curricula, policies, and reports; maintaining an online database of projects funded by the HRSA and MCHB; and responding to information requests on topics such as early childhood caries, dental sealants, fluoride varnish, and access to and reimbursement for oral health services [39].

The Bureau of Primary Health Care (BPHC) provides national leadership in assessing the nation's health care needs of underserved populations and in assisting communities to provide primary health care services to the underserved to help eliminate health disparities. The BPHC provides support to community health centers that provide primary services to rural and medically underserved populations in spite of their ability to pay. They form a major component of the "safety net" system. In 2006, BPHC grantees had 6,250 FTE health professionals who provided 6,149,694 encounters for 2,557,003 patients [39]. Community Health Centers that receive federal grant subsidy as a primary means of funding are referred to as federally qualified health centers (FQHC). All new FQHCs are required to assure access to oral health services [40].

Seventy-three percent of existing federally-funded health centers provided oral health services onsite, as compared with 34% in 1997. Others referred patients to contracted private providers. Dental visits constituted about 10% of all visits to the federally-funded health centers in 2005, a growth of 87% since 2000 [41].

The Migrant Health Program supports the delivery of migrant health services that includes dental services with other prevention-oriented and pediatric services. These programs serve over 650,000 migrant and seasonal farm workers. In 2002, 85.1% (103) of 121 Migrant Health Programs provided some type of dental care [10].

The Bureau of Health Professions (BHPr) coordinates, evaluates, and supports the development and use of the nation's health personnel [42]. The BHPr has defined the public health dental worker as the individual who "...plans, develops, implements and evaluates dental health programs to promote and maintain optimum oral health of the public" [43]. Many of these individuals work in a public health program, such as community health centers where clinical services or dental treatment is provided to high risk or vulnerable populations. They may or may not have formal training in public health. This includes dental professionals, such as dentists, dental hygienists, dental assistants, dental technicians, and other personnel.

A Health Professional Shortage Area (HPSA) is a geographic area, population group, or health care facility that has been designated by the federal government as having a shortage of health professionals. Vulnerable population groups bear a disproportionately heavier burden of oral disease. The purpose of the HPSA designation is to reverse the unequal oral disease and access challenge.

There are three categories of HPSAs: primary care, dental, and mental health. HPSAs are designated using several criteria, including population-to-clinician ratios. This ratio is usually 3,500 to 1 for primary care, 5,000 to 1 for dental care, and 30,000 to 1 for mental health care. HPSAs are assigned a numerical score from 1 to 26 based on the level of need. The higher score has greater priority. The number of dental HPSAs (DHPSA) has steadily increased, from 805 in 1991 to 3,724 in 2007, affecting about 48 million people in these areas. The number of additional practitioners needed to remove a DHPSA designation is 6,701 dentists, and 9,318 are needed to meet target ratios. Thirty-four percent of these areas are in metropolitan areas and the rest are in nonmetropolitan areas [44].

National Health Service Corps

This HRSA program is managed through the BHPr and provides incentives to health professionals to work in communities that would otherwise be without health care. Some of the strategies adopted by the National Health Service Corps (NHSC) are forming partnerships with communities and organizations, student loan repayment, and recruiting culturally competent clinicians [45]. The NHSC program has a field strength of more than 4,000 clinicians and health care professionals who provide care to over 4 million people nationwide. About half of these are in community health centers. The field strength for dentists in 2006 was 415, and 42 for dental hygienists [46]. Currently, the NHSC uses loan repayment as the main incentive to attract professionals to work with underserved populations.

Other federal departments also have programs that provide oral health services; these include the US Departments of Defense, Transportation, and Veterans Affairs. The US Department of Agriculture administers the Women, Infants, and Children program that increasingly serves as a link for prevention, early detection, and referral of early childhood tooth decay in high-risk children [47].

State dental public health infrastructure and oral health programs

Each state's Department of Health is very important for improving the oral health of the populations they serve. Most states have a dental director who coordinates efforts and helps ensure that necessary programs and services are provided. These may include, but are not limited to programs for the following [10]:

- Access to oral health services and workforce studies
- Early Childhood Caries (formerly Baby Bottle Tooth Decay)
- Fluoridation advocacy
- School fluoride mouth rinse and dental sealants
- Fluoride supplements and fluoride varnish
- Mouth guard and injury prevention
- Clinical services and infection control
- Dental screening, needs assessment, and oral health surveys
- Oral health education and promotion
- Smoke and spit tobacco cessation
- Water fluoridation monitoring and private well fluoride testing
- Prevent Abuse and Neglect through Dental Awareness (PANDA)

State dental directors may be full-time or part-time. There is considerable variation in the professional training and academic qualification of these directors. As of 2007, 44 states had a full-time state dental director position [48]. Of the filled positions, there were 29 dentists and 9 dental hygienists. Of the 29 dentists, 21 had a Masters in Public Health (MPH) degree and one had a Juris Doctor degree. Three of the dental directors who are dental hygienists had an MPH degree and one had a doctorate. Seven states had vacant positions, yet to be filled. (Dean Perkins, DDS, MPH, Executive Director Association of States and Territorial Directors, personal communication, September, 2007). In 2002, the median number of FTEs in state dental programs was three and the range was 0 to 81 [10]. The budget for dental activities in different states in 2001 and 2002 ranged from less $100,000 to over $1,000,000. In 2002, 5.9% of the states spent less than $100,000 and 35% of the states spent over $1,000,000 (Table 1).

Local health department infrastructure and oral health programs

The local health departments (LHDs) in the cities, towns and counties of the United States are the building block of a functioning public health infrastructure. They are defined as an administrative or service unit of local or state government concerned with health, and carrying some responsibility for the health of a jurisdiction smaller than the state [49]. The LHDs are meant to understand the unique health problems facing their communities and develop programs and policies to meet these needs. They are guided by a set of regulations that ensure they offer services to improve the health of their jurisdiction. In 2005, there were 2,864 LHDs in the United States. Rhode Island is the only state without an LHD. All of these health departments are unique in their size, activities, jurisdiction, and infrastructure [48].

In the 2005's National Profile of Local Health Department Reports, oral health services were directly provided by the LHD in 31% of those surveyed,

Table 1
Budgets for state dental public health programs 2001, 2002

Total budget for states for dental public health programs	2001		2002	
	Number of states	Percentage of states responding (%)	Number of states	Percentage of states responding (%)
<$100,000	4	8.9	2	5.9
$100,000–$250,000	7	15.6	7	20.6
$250,001–$500,000	7	15.6	5	14.7
$500,001–1,000,000	13	28.9	8	23.5
≥$1,000,000	14	31.1	12	35.3
Total	45	100	34	100

2001 and 2002 State Synopsis Surveys of Dental Public Health Programs conducted by the Association of State and Territorial Dental Directors and the Centers for Disease Control and Prevention, Division of Oral Health.

Data from Tomar SL. Assessment of the dental public health infrastructure in the United States. National Institute of Dental and Craniofacial Research, 2004. Available at: http://www.nidcr.nih. gov/NewsAndReports/ReportsPresentation/Executive_Summary_Assesment_Dental. Accessed July 2007.

and by nongovernmental organizations in 55% [50]. The funding for these has been from local sources (29%), directly by the state (23%), and federal funds to LHDs through state agencies (13%). One-third of LHDs have annual expenditures of under $500,000, and one-fifth are over $5 million. The median LHD per capita annual expenditure (excluding clinical service revenue) is $23. There have been many local and community attempts to incorporate oral health into the essential public services. These initiatives address issues, such as building community coalitions, and starting community oral health programs, such as safety-net dental clinics, mobile dental clinics, and school-based prevention and sealant programs [51–53]. Some of the larger dental programs have been in cities and counties like Alameda County in California, Birmingham, Boston, Cincinnati, Multnomah County in Oregon, New York City, Seattle-King County in Washington State, and West Palm Beach.

Community health centers that do not receive any subsidy from the federal government may also be locally funded, with LHDs playing a key role. Although no accurate data is available, there are estimated to be one and a half times more health centers than the FQHCs, with approximately 904 of these health centers providing dental care. Limited funding in the non-FQHC may translate into having fewer full-time personnel and seeing fewer patients than the FQHCs. Many of these programs were initiated, supported, or funded by local and county health departments.

Dental public health organizations

There are a number of professional and advocacy public health and dental organizations that promote oral health. They all play an important role in providing information and resources to the dental public health work-force, the dental profession, and the public (Appendix 1) [54].

American Public Health Association, Oral Health Section

The American Public Health Association (APHA), founded in 1872, is the oldest and largest public health association in the world. It is also the Secretariat for the World Federation of Public Health Associations and publishes the *American Journal of Public Health*. As APHA is a multidisci plinary public health association, it provides its dental public health members with a forum to obtain support for oral health programs and initiatives from nondental public health leaders and decision-makers.

The Oral Health Section in APHA investigates and promotes cutting edge oral health issues that are in the publics' interest. These include access to dental care for vulnerable populations, dentistry in a national health program, community water fluoridation, reducing racial and ethnic disparities in health, domestic violence screening, identification and referral by dental health professionals, dental sealants, and preventing the transmission of blood borne pathogens, to name a few [55].

American Association of Public Health Dentistry

The American Association of Public Health Dentistry (AAPHD) began in 1937 and strives to improve oral health through promotion of effective efforts in disease prevention, health promotion, and service delivery; education of the public, health professionals, and decision-makers regarding the importance of oral health to total well-being; and expansion of the knowledge base of dental public health and fostering competency in its practice [56].

The AAPHD started as a group of state dental directors with restricted membership. Since then the membership criteria has been broadened to include any one working to improve oral health [57]. The AAPHD is the sponsor of the American Board of Public Health, publishes the *Journal of Public Health Dentistry,* and is a cosponsor of the yearly National Oral Health Conference with the Association of State and Territorial Dental Directors (ASTDD).

American Board of Dental Public Health

The American Board of Dental Public Health (ABDPH) is a not-for-profit organization incorporated in 1950, and is the national examining and certifying agency for the specialty of dental public health. The Board was organized in accordance with the Requirements for Approval of Examining Boards in Dental Specialties of the ADAs Council on Dental Education and Licensure [58].

The principal purposes of the Board, as defined in its Articles of Incorporation, are to protect and improve the public's health by the study and creation of standards for the practice of dental public health; grant and issue dental public health certificates to dentists who have successfully completed the prescribed training and experience requisite for the practice of dental public health; and ensure continuing competency of diplomates.

Association of State and Territorial Dental Directors

The ASTDD is primarily made up of state dental directors and provides information and advocacy to the states and territories in the United States. The ASTDD supports programs and initiatives for community water fluoridation, school fluoride programs, school sealant programs, workforce development, special health care needs, and access to oral health services, which may include services to special groups such as adults and seniors. The ASTDD helps develop state oral health surveillance systems, state oral health coalition, and oral health plans, and promotes best practices for state, territorial, and community oral health programs. The ASTDD is also an important resource in meeting the oral health objectives of Healthy People 2010 and the National Call to Action to Promote Oral Health.

American Association of Community Dental Programs

The American Association of Community Dental Programs (AACDP) supports the efforts of those with an interest in serving the oral health needs at the community level. Members include local dental directors and staff of city, county, and community-based health programs [59]. The AACDP developed two publications to help local public health agencies incorporate oral health into public health services. These are *A Guide for Developing and Enhancing Community Oral Health Programs* and *A Model Framework for Community Oral Health Programs Based Upon the Ten Essential Public Health Services.*

American Dental Education Association

The mission of the American Dental Education Association (ADEA) is to lead individuals and institutions of the dental education community to address contemporary issues influencing education, research, and the delivery of oral health care for the improvement of the health of the public. The ADEA has a section on community and preventive dentistry and behavioral sciences. The ADEA publishes the *Journal of Dental Education* and the *Bulletin of Dental Education.*

National Network on Oral Health Access

The National Network on Oral Health Access is a nationwide network of dental providers who care for patients in Migrant, Homeless, and Community Health Centers. Members have displayed commitment to improving the health of the underserved through increased access to oral health services [60].

Summary

Dental public health is a unique and challenging specialty because the patient being served is an entire population or community, rather than just an individual patient. This population may be a school, neighborhood, nursing home, town, city, state, or nation, or a combination of these different communities. A high priority is also given to vulnerable or high risk populations, such as children, the elderly, low income, developmentally disabled, homebound, homeless, persons with HIV/AIDS, the underserved, and minorities. The primary emphasis of dental public health is prevention and organized community efforts. Education and training in epidemiology, biostatistics, policy, management administration, and research are key for the dental public health professional. Unfortunately, there are only 155 active board-certified dentists in dental public health, but 2,032 dentists in the United States who work in public health, of which 1,000 have at least 1 year of advanced education beyond dental school; over 600 have 2 years of advanced education beyond dental school. Public health dentists and hygienists maximize limited resources to meet a great, unmet dental need. The dental public health infrastructure works in government at the local, state, and national level, as well as in organizations and institutions. Dental public health professionals play a key role in influencing policy and programs that affect the quality of life of millions of people every day.

Appendix 1

Web resources for dental public health organizations

Organization and Web site	Link/resources available
American Association of Public Health Dentistry (AAPHD)	www.aaphd.org
American Dental Education Association (ADEA)	http://www.adea.org/
	www.explorehealthcareers.org/en/index.asp
	Managed by ADEA, this Web site provides information on healthcare career opportunities for underrepresented minorities.
Association of State and Territorial Dental Directors (ASTDD)	www.astdd.org
	www.astdd.org/docs/astddguidelines_bestpraclinksmay 2005rev7final6.29.2005.pdf
	Provides guidelines and best practices for states and territorial oral health programs.
American Association of Community Dental Programs (AACDP)	www.aacdp.com
	www.mchoralhealth.org/Seal
	Seal America: The Prevention Invention
	http://www.mobile-portabledentalmanual.com/
	Mobile Dental Programs
	www.aacdp.com/guide/appendixE.html
	A guide for developing and enhancing community oral health programs
	www.aacdp.com/Docs/Framework.pdf.
	A model framework for community oral health programs based upon the Ten Essential Public Health Services

(continued on next page)

Organization and Web site	Link/resources available
American Public Health Association, Oral Health Section	www.apha-oh.org
Centers for Disease Control and Prevention (CDC)/Oral Health	www.cdc.gov/oralhealth
American Board of Dental Public Health	www.aaphd.org/default.asp?page=ABDPHMenu.htm
Health Resources and Services Administration (HRSA)	www.hrsa.hhs.gov
	Bureaus active in oral health include:
	HIV Bureau
	http://hab.hrsa.gov
	Bureau of Health Professions
	http://bhpr.hrsa.gov/
	Bureau of Primary Care
	http://bphc.hrsa.gov/
	Bureau of Maternal and Child Health
	http://mchb.hrsa.gov/
	National Maternal and Child Oral Health Resource Center
	www.mchoralhealth.org
	www.mchlibrary.info/KnowledgePaths/ kp_oralhealth.html
	Knowledge Path: Oral Health and Children and Adolescent, an electronic guide of resources aimed at improving access to and the quality of oral health services for children and adolescents.
National Oral Health Policy Center	www.healthychild.ucla.edu/nohpc/Default.asp
	Provides relevant information and data on access to oral health care
National Institute of Dental and Craniofacial Research (NIDCR)	www.nidcr.nih.gov/
National Association of County and City Health Officials (NACCHO)	www.naccho.org
	www.naccho.org/topics/infrastructure/ operational_definition.cfm
	Operational definition of a local public health agency
National Network for Oral health Access (NNOHA)	www.nnoha.org

Data from Tomar SL. An assessment of the dental public health infrastructure in the United States. J Public Health Dent 2006;66(1):3–4.

References

[1] Allukian M. The neglected epidemic and the Surgeon General's Report: a call to action for better oral health [editorial]. Am J Public Health 2000;90(6):843–5.
[2] Competency Statement for Dental Public Health. American Association Public Health Dentistry (AAPHD). Available at: http://www.aaphd.org/default.asp?page=competencies.htm. Accessed August 6, 2007.

[3] Report of ADA Recognized Dental Specialty Certifying Boards. Council on Dental Education and Licensure. Chicago: American Dental Association; 2007.

[4] Tomar LS. An assessment of the dental public health infrastructure in the United States. J Public Health Dent 2006;66(1):5–16.

[5] Preamble to the competency statements for Dental Public Health. J Public Health Dent 1998; 58(1):119–24.

[6] The United States Health Workforce Profile, October 2006. The New York Center for Health Work Force Studies.

[7] U.S. Department of Health and Human Services. Public Health Workforce Report, Health Resources and Services Administration. Bureau of Health Professions January 2005, 19–22.

[8] Valachovic RW, Weaver RG, Sinkford JC, et al. Trends in dentistry and dental education. J Dent Educ 2001;6:539–61.

[9] 2004 Dental Education at a Glance, American Dental Education Association (ADEA). Available at: http://www.adea.org/DEPR/2004_Dental_Ed_At_A_Glance.pdf. Accessed September 7, 2007.

[10] Tomar LS. National Institute of Dental and Craniofacial Research (NIDCR) Assessment of the Dental Public Health Infrastructure in the United States. 2004. Available at: http://www.nidcr.nih.cov/NR/rdonlyres/A981AOlCD437/O/USDentalPublicHealthInfrastructure 82004.pdf. Accessed July 2007.

[11] Mckinnon M, Luke G, Bresch J, et al. Emerging Allied Dental Workforce Models: considerations for academic medical institutions. J Dent Educ 2007;77(11):1476–91.

[12] U.S. Department of Health and Human Services. Oral Health in America: a Report of the Surgeon General. Rockville (MD): U.S. Department of Health and Human Services, National Institute of Dental and Craniofacial Research, National Institutes of Health; 2000.

[13] FY 2008 Budget in Brief, The Department of Health and Human Services. Available at: http://www.hhs.gov/budget/08budget/2008BudgetInBrief.pdf. Accessed November 10, 2007.

[14] Office of the Assistant Secretary of Health, Office of the Surgeon General. Final Report to the House of Representatives, Appropriations Committee on Oral Health Activities, Department of Health and Human Services. May 1989.

[15] Improving the Oral Health of American People Opportunity for Action. A Study of the Oral Health Activities of the Department of Health and Human Services, Interim Study Group Activities March 1989.

[16] Healthy People 2010. Available at: www.HealthyPeople.Gov. Accessed December 17, 2007.

[17] U.S. Public Health Service Report to the Council on Access, Prevention and Interprofessional Relations (CAPIR), American Dental Association, September 2006.

[18] Introduction to Indian Health Service Indian Health Service (IHS). Available at: http://www.ihs.gov/PublicInfo/PublicAffairs/Welcome_Info/IHSintro.asp. Accessed November 28, 2007.

[19] Sekiguchi E, Guay AH, Jackson Brown L, et al. Improving oral health care of Alaska natives. Am J Public Health 2005;95:769–73.

[20] U.S. Public Health Service Report to the Council on Access, Prevention and Interprofessional Relations (CAPIR), American Dental Association, February 2007.

[21] Indian Health Service Workforce IHS. Available at: http://info.ihs.gov/files/workforce-Jan2007.doc. Accessed September 27, 2007.

[22] Budget Request Summary Fiscal Year 2008. Centers for Disease Control and Prevention. (CDC) February 2007. Available at: http://www.cdc.gov/fmo/PDFs/FY08_Budget_Summary_Final.pdf. Accessed September 1, 2007.

[23] Overview of the Oral Health Division, Centers for Disease Control and Prevention CDC U.S. Public Health Service Report to the Council on Access, Prevention and Interprofessional Relations (CAPIR), American Dental Association, August 2007.

[24] About NIDCR National Institute for Dental and Craniofacial Research. Available at: http://www.nidcr.nih.gov/AboutNIDCR/MissionStatement.htm. Accessed August 29, 2007.

[25] Research Sponsored by National Institute for Dental and Craniofacial Research. Available at: http://www.nidcr.nih.gov/Research/Extramural/DER.htm. Accessed August 30, 2007.

[26] NIDCR Report, U.S. Public Health Service Report to the Council on Access, Prevention and Interprofessional Relations (CAPIR), American Dental Association, August 2007.

[27] Dental Coverage and Care for Low Income Children: A Role for Medicaid and SCHIP. The Kaiser Commission on Medicaid and the Uninsured, August 2007. Available at: http://www.kff.org/medicaid/upload/7681.pdf. Accessed September 6, 2007.

[28] National Health Expenditure Data, Center for Medicare and Medicaid Services (CMS), Office of the Actuary. Available at: http://www.cms.hhs.gov/NationalHealthExpendData/downloads/nhe2005.zip. Accessed August 3, 2007.

[29] U.S. Census Bureau. Health insurance: coverage 2006 highlights. Available at: http://www.census.gov/hhes/www/hlthins/hlthin06/hlth06asc.html. Accessed September 2007.

[30] Manski RJ, Brown E. Dental Use, Expenses, Private Dental Coverage, and Changes, 1996 and 2004. Rockville (MD):Agency for Healthcare Research and Quality; 2007. MEPS Chartbook No.17. Available at: http://www.meps.ahrq.gov/mepsweb/data_files/publications/cb17/cb17.pdf.

[31] U.S Census Bureau Income, Poverty, and Health Insurance Coverage in the United States: 2006 Current Population Reports August 2007. Available at: http://www.census.gov/prod/2007pubs/p60-233.pdf. Accessed September 27, 2007.

[32] Overview of Medicare Dental Coverage. Center for Medicare and Medicaid Services. (CMS). Available at: http://www.cms.hhs.gov/MedicareDentalCoverage/. Accessed September 27, 2007.

[33] Mertz E, O'Neil E. The growing challenge of providing oral health care services to all Americans. Health Aff 2002;21(5):65–77.

[34] Coughlin TA, Long SK, Shen Y, et al. Assessing access to care under Medicaid: Evidence for the Nation and Thirteen States. Health Aff 2005;24:1073–83.

[35] HRSA Overview. Available at: http://www.hrsa.gov/about/default.htm. Accessed August 25, 2007.

[36] MCHB Oral Health Objectives Programs. Available at: http://mchb.hrsa.gov/programs/default.htm. Accessed September 29, 2007.

[37] About Oral Health Policy Center, UCLA Center for healthier children, families and communities. http://www.healthychild.ucla.edu/nohpc/Default.asp. Accessed October 1, 2007.

[38] About National Maternal and Child Oral Health Resource Center. http://www.mchoralhealth.org/about.html. Accessed September 29, 2007.

[39] Uniform Data System UDS, Health Resources and Services Administration. http://bphc.hrsa.gov/uds/2006data/national/nationaltable2.htm. Accessed October, 2007.

[40] Health Center Program Expectations Bureau of Primary Health Care (BPHC) Policy Information Notice: 98–23. August 17, 1998. Available at: ftp://ftp.hrsa.gov/bphc/docs/1998PINS/PIN98-23.PDF. Accessed September 1, 2007.

[41] Rudy G. Health centers role in addressing the oral health needs of the medically underserved. August 2007 National Association of Community Health Center. http://www.nachc.com/research/Files/Oral%20Health%20Report%20FINAL.pdf. Accessed September 8, 2007.

[42] Mission of Bureau of Health Professions. Available at: http://bhpr.hrsa.gov/. Accessed September 24, 2007.

[43] Bureau of Health Professions, National Center for Health Workforce Information and Analysis. The Public Health Workforce 2000. http//www.nursing.columbia.edu/chphsr/pdf/enum2000.pdf. Accessed August 15, 2007.

[44] Selected Statistics on Health Professional Shortage Areas As of June 30, 2007, Shortage Designation Branch, Office of Workforce Evaluation and Quality and Assurance, Bureau of Health Professions, HRSA.

[45] The National Health Service Corp (NHSC) Mission. http://nhsc.bhpr.hrsa.gov/about/mission.asp. Accessed September 23, 2007.

[46] U.S. Department of Health and Human Services. Healthy people 2010: understanding and improving health. In: U.S. Department of Health and Human Services. 2nd edition. Washington, DC: U.S. Government Printing Office; 2000.

[47] Healthy People 2010 Oral Health Toolkit, National Institute for Dental and Craniofacial Research. NIDCR. Available at: http://www.nidcr.nih.gov/NewsAndReports/ ReportsPresentation/HealthyPeople/Chapter2.htm. Accessed October 2, 2007.

[48] Activities and Workforce of Small Town Rural Local Health Departments. Findings from the 2005 National Profile of Local Health Departments Study, May 2007 (NACCHO). Available at: http://www.naccho.org/topics/infrastructure/documents/LHD_Rural_final. pdf. Accessed September 22, 2007.

[49] Operational definition of a local public health agency (NACCHO). Available at: http:// www.naccho.org/topics/infrastructure/operational_definition.cfm. Accessed September 2007.

[50] 2005 National Profile of Local Health Departments, July 2006. Available at: http://www. naccho.org/topics/infrastructure/documents/NACCHO_report_final_000.pdf. Accessed September 22, 2007.

[51] Cohen LA, Horowitz AM. Community-Based Sealant programs in the United States: Results of a survey, JPHD, 50:6, pp.406-417 Spec. Issue, 1990.

[52] Safety Net Dental Clinic Manual. Available at: http://www.dentalclinicmanual.com/ doc_download/safetynet_usersguide.pdf. Accessed June 20, 2007.

[53] Mobile Dental Clinic Manual. Available at: http://www.mobile-portabledentalmanual.com/. Accessed July 12, 2007.

[54] King R. Healthy People 2010 oral health objectives—the role of AAPHD. J Public Health Dent 2001;61(4):195–6.

[55] About Oral Health Section, American Public Health Association (APHA). Available at: http://www.apha-oh.org/about.htm. Accessed September 23, 2007.

[56] About AAPHD, American Association of Public Health Dentistry. Available at: http:// www.aaphd.org/default.asp?page=about.htm. Accessed September 12, 2007.

[57] Striffler DF. A Historical Review of the American Association of Public Health Dentists, Prepared for presentation at the AAPHD Planning Workshop, July 18 – 20, 1978, Atlanta Georgia.

[58] American Board of Dental Public Health Incorporated Informational Brochure Revised 2007. Available at: http://www.aaphd.org/default.asp?page=ABDPHMenu.htm. Accessed September 14, 2007.

[59] About American Association of Community Dental Program (AACDP). Available at: http://www.aacdp.com/. Accessed September 27, 2007.

[60] About National Network on Oral Health Access NNOHA. Available at: http://www.nnoha. org/index.htm. Accessed November 26, 2007.

ELSEVIER
SAUNDERS

THE DENTAL
CLINICS
OF NORTH AMERICA

Dent Clin N Am 52 (2008) 281–295

Financing Dental Care: Trends in Public and Private Expenditures for Dental Services

Howard Bailit, DMD, PhD[a],*, Tryfon Beazoglou, PhD[b]

[a]Department of Community Medicine, School of Medicine, University of Connecticut,
263 Farmington Avenue, Farmington, CT 06030-6325, USA
[b]Department of Craniofacial Sciences, School of Dental Medicine, University of Connecticut,
263 Farmington Avenue, Farmington, CT 06030-1610, USA

The financing of dental care is concerned with the amount and sources of funds that pay for personal dental services. These monies are paid to dental practices and clinics for the services provided to patients. They do not include the monies allocated for community level dental public health programs such as water fluoridation and public education. Although the exact percentages are not known, probably 90% or more of national dental expenditures go to pay for personal dental services [1].

The amount and sources of funds that are spent on dental care are important for several reasons. First, the amount of money spent on dental care is an indication of the population's access to dental services and their oral health status. The United States spends much more money on a per capita basis for personal dental services than most other developed countries, which is one reason why the oral health status of Americans is better than in most developed countries [2]. There are significant differences in dental expenditures among population subgroups within the United States. As is well known, low income families spend much less money on dental care than high income families, and this difference explains, in large part, the substantial disparities in access to care and oral health seen in this country [3].

Second, the source of funds is important, because payers have a major say on the amount of money allocated for dental services and how the money is spent. Employers, government, and individual patients are the primary payers for dental services. For privately insured patients, employers

* Corresponding author.
E-mail address: bailit@nso1.uchc.edu (H. Bailit).

are the main payers for care, and they usually contract with insurers to administer these funds. As the primary payer, employers have a major role in deciding how much money is spent on dental benefits and how these costs will be shared with employees. In general, large employers spend much more money on dental benefits than do small employers. The richness of the dental benefit plan is a major determinant of how often patients seek dental care and the services that they receive when they go to dentists [4].

Working through insurers, payers also decide what services are covered benefits, the amount and types of patient cost-sharing for the covered services, and how dentists are paid for their services. Practicing dentists have to be concerned with these financing issues because they influence dentists' incomes and the services patients receive.

To address these important issues, this article first considers trends in total expenditures for dental care and compares the growth of dental expenditures with that of other common health care services. The sources of these funds are then described, followed by an examination of the factors that explain the growth of dental expenditures. Within each topic area, the health policy implications are considered, especially as they impact private dental practitioners. The article ends with a general discussion of these trends and their influence on access to dental care and dentist's incomes.

Total expenditures

As shown in Fig. 1, $86.6 billion was spent on personal dental services in 2005, 5.5 times more dollars than in 1980 [1]. Relative to total national spending for all health care, dental treatment accounts for 4.4%. Although this percentage may seem like a small amount of money, it is not. For example, $83.6 billion dollars is spent annually (2007) to treat coronary heart disease [6] and $74 billion to treat cancer (2005) [7]. In terms of these

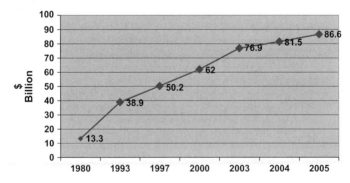

Fig. 1. National expenditures for personal dental services, selected years, 1980 to 2005. (*Data from* Center for Medicare and Medicaid Services. National health expenditures aggregate amounts and average annual percent change, by type of expenditure: selected calendar years 1960–2005. Available at: http://www.cms.hhs.gov/NationalHealthExpendData/downloads/tables.pdf. Accessed July 2007.)

comparisons, expenditures for dental care are substantial. The difference is that relatively few people receive care for heart disease or cancer, but over half the population receives dental care each year.

Over this 25-year time period, the average annual increase in dental expenditures was 7.2%, more than twice the annual rate of general inflation (3.2%) [1]. The Center for Medicare and Medicaid Services, a federal agency, projects that the growth of dental expenditures will slow down somewhat for the next 6 years, reaching $126.3 billion in 2013 [8]. This growth is an increase of almost $40 billion, with an average annual growth of 6.6%.

Table 1 compares the growth in expenditures for dental services versus the costs for physicians, hospitals, prescription drugs, nursing homes, and total expenditures [1]. Overall, expenditures for the other medical services grew faster than that for dental services. Costs for prescription drugs led the group, with an average annual increase of about 11.9%. Although expenditures for dental care are increasing faster than the general economy, the rate of increase is less than for other medical services. This difference explains why the percentage of total health dollars spent on dental care is declining each year.

Policy implications

Of considerable interest is the slow down in spending for physicians and hospitals but not dentists in 1997 and 2000 [1]. This reduction was due to the impact of managed care on physician and hospital expenditures. Managed care had little impact on dental care expenditures for several reasons. First, managed care is a type of insurance plan, and fewer Americans have private dental insurance when compared with those who have private medical insurance. Without dental insurance, there is no managed care. Second, dental insurance plans require substantial patient cost-sharing (eg, deductibles and co-insurance) when compared with medical plans; therefore, patient

Table 1

National health expenditures, average annual percent growth from prior year for selected years and average over all years, 1980 to 2005

Spending category	Average annual percent growth from prior year						Average, 1980–2005 (%)
	1980	1993	1997	2000	2003	2005	
Dentists	11.1	8.6	6.6	7.3	7.4	6.3	7.2
Physicians	12.9	11.8	4.6	6.2	8.3	7.0	9.2
Hospitals	13.9	9.2	3.6	4.6	8.0	7.9	7.5
Prescription drugs	8.2	11.7	11.1	15.9	13.1	5.8	11.9
Nursing homes	16.8	10.0	6.6	4.1	5.1	6.0	7.7
Total	13.1	10.3	5.5	5.9	8.3	7.1	8.6

Data from Center for Medicare and Medicaid Services. National health expenditures aggregate amounts and average annual percent change, by type of expenditure: selected calendar years 1960–2005. Available at: http://www.cms.hhs.gov/NationalHealthExpendData/downloads/tables.pdf. Accessed July 2007.

cost-sharing is already a significant barrier to increased expenditures, and there is relatively little to gain by the traditional cost-control techniques used in managed care. Third, insurance companies have much less negotiating leverage with dentists when compared with physicians, because the number of dentists relative to the size of the population is declining, which is not true for physicians. Also, dental insurers have, on average, much less market share in a given geographic location than medical insurers. The latter two facts mean that dentists do not have to join managed care plans to have an adequate supply of patients. In fact, less than 50% of dentists participate in a managed care plan. In contrast, almost 90% of physicians are enrolled in managed care plans [9].

In 2003 and 2006, the monies spent on physicians and hospitals substantially increased, suggesting that the impact of managed care was limited to a brief time period and, currently, is not effective in controlling the rate of increase in health care expenditures. The bottom line is that aggregate expenditures for personal health services continue to grow almost three times faster than general inflation.

This rate of growth in health care costs is not sustainable in the long run because payers (businesses, government, and individuals) have to take funds from other priority areas and reallocate them to health care. For government, this means spending less for programs such as public education, research, and roads. For individuals, this means spending less for housing, vacations, and other things. The alternative to spending more money is to reduce the amount and types of services available to patients. In fact, both things are happening. Indeed, almost 20% of our national wealth is directed toward paying for health care services [1]. At the same time, the rapid growth of health care costs is the primary reason why almost 47 million Americans under the age of 65 years (15% of this population) are not covered by health insurance at any one point in time [10]. Clearly, these issues are explosive political topics, and the control of health care costs is certain to dominate domestic politics for the next 10 or more years. Whatever steps are taken to control increases in health care costs, they are certain to have a significant impact on the practice of medicine and possibly dentistry.

Assuming that the solution to the problem of rapidly rising costs and uninsured patients is some form of government regulation of medical care finances, the key question is whether dentistry will be included in the government plan. In some countries, dental care is included in the national health plan, whereas in others it is not [11]. In the United States, there is a good possibility that dental care for children will be an integral part of the plan but not adult care.

Payment sources

Table 2 gives expenditures for selected personal health services by fund source in 2005 [1]. The two main fund sources are private and public.

Table 2
Expenditures for personal health care by type of service and source of funds, 2005

Category	Expenditures in billions of US dollars						
	Total	Out-of-pocket	Private health insurance	Total	Medicare	Medicaid	Other
Dental	81.4	38.3	43.1	5.2	0.1	4.5	0.6
Physicians	272.7	42.5	203.3	148.5	89.3	30.3	28.9
Hospitals	264.5	20.1	217.0	347.1	180.3	106.3	60.5
Prescription drugs	146.1	50.9	95.2	54.6	4.0	37.6	13.0
Nursing homes	57.9	37.4	9.1	75.9	19.2	53.5	3.3
Total	914.5	249.4	596.7	746.9	331.4	302.2	113.3

Data from Center for Medicare and Medicaid Services. National health expenditures aggregate amounts and average annual percent change, by type of expenditure: selected calendar years 1960–2005. Available at: http://www.cms.hhs.gov/NationalHealthExpendData/downloads/tables.pdf. Accessed July 2007.

Almost all dental services are paid for from private funding sources ($81.4 billion), namely, private insurance and patients (out-of-pocket). Only 6% ($5.2 billion) comes from a public fund, the Medicaid program that pays for the care of some 30 million low income Americans. The Medicare program for elderly Americans provides little dental coverage (only when dental care is an integral part of treating a medical problem).

This limited commitment of public funds for dental care is in contrast to that for most other medical services. For example, federal and state governments pay for 57% of hospital care, 35% of physician services, and 62% of nursing home care. These allocations of public funds indicate that access to dental care has a relatively low priority in government health plans.

The two primary sources of private dental funds are employer-based insurance and individuals paying for care out-of-pocket. Of these sources, employer insurance pays for 52.9%. This percentage is very high considering that only one third of the population is covered by an employer-based dental insurance plan. People with private dental insurance receive a lot more care when compared with those without this benefit [4].

The remaining private expenditures come from insured patients who have to pay deductibles and co-insurance for covered services (and the total amount for uncovered services) and from patients without insurance who have to pay for all services out-of-pocket. In contrast, private payments to physicians and hospitals come overwhelmingly from private insurance. Private insurance covers 85% of private funds paid to physicians and 93% of private funds paid to hospitals.

Another way to look at this issue is to compare total out-of-pocket expenditures versus private and public insurance. From this perspective, people pay out-of-pocket for 44.2% of dental care, 10.1% of physician services, and 3.0% of hospital care. This stark contrast indicates why the general population perceives dental care to be so expensive [12]. The fact is that they are paying much more out-of-pocket for dental care when compared with care from physicians and hospitals even though total expenditures for dental care are only a small percentage of these other services.

Policy implications

Actually, the out-of-pocket dental expenses of privately insured patients are considerably higher than these numbers suggest because most employers require employees to contribute to dental insurance premiums. In fact, for the average family plan, employees pay about 70% of the premiums with before tax dollars [13]. Employers pay the other 30%. Although private insurance pays for 30% of privately funded dental care, employees contribute a large percentage of these funds. If employee contributions to premiums are added to patient payments for deductibles and co-insurance, many employees are financially better off without dental insurance. That is, they are paying more for dental care with insurance than without it. This issue becomes significant when employers make dental insurance an optional benefit. Many employees who are in good oral health or who have small families opt not to enroll in dental plans. Those selecting dental insurance often have families that expect to use a lot of care. From an insurance perspective, this causes dental premiums to increase rapidly because more plan participants are heavy users of dental services. In the long run, fewer employees will select dental benefits because high premiums will further exacerbate the problem. Employees' contributions to premiums are paid with before tax dollars, which is an indirect type of government subsidy. Without this subsidy, few employees would enroll in employer-based dental insurance plans.

Because private dental insurance is a major driver of patient use of services and, in turn, dentists' incomes, trends in the number of people with dental insurance are an important issue. The data that are available (Fig. 2) indicate that, surprisingly, the percentage of full- and part-time

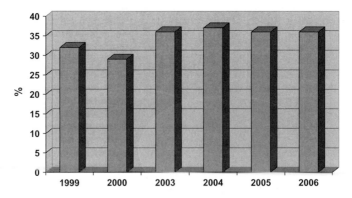

Fig. 2. Percentage of all private industry workers participating in dental care benefit plans, 1999 to 2006. (*Data from* US Department of Labor. Bureau of Labor Statistics. Percent of all workers participating in dental care benefits, all private industry, 1999–2006. Available at: http://data.bls.gov/. Accessed July 2007.)

employees with private dental insurance has increased modestly from 32% in 1999 to 36% in 2006 [14]. For just full-time workers, the percentage is even higher, 44% (2006). This increase is surprising because the percentage of employees with private medical insurance is declining, and the number of people without medical insurance is growing [15]. The stability of private dental insurance enrollment probably results from this benefit mainly being offered by large employers and the fact that, thus far, most large employers have not eliminated dental benefits. In contrast, many small companies are dropping medical insurance benefits or making the employee contribution to premiums so large that many employees decline enrollment. Instead of dropping dental insurance, many large employers appear to be passing on most of the cost of premiums to employees.

Low income families

Because of national concerns with access disparities, the financing of dental care for lower income populations deserves special attention. Approximately 92.5 million people out of almost 300 million Americans (30.8%) are considered to have low incomes (2000) [3]. This classification is defined as an income below 200% of the Federal Poverty Level. As seen in Table 3, 22.9% of the low income population in the year 2000 visited the dentist one or more times compared with 36.5% of middle income and 56.5% of high income families [3]. There are major differences among family income groups in their access to dental services.

Table 3 also gives the mean expense per person with a visit and the sources of payment by family income group [3]. In terms of expenditures for those persons visiting a dentist, the low income group average is substantially lower ($395) than the average for middle ($467) and high ($529) income groups. For payment sources, the percent out-of-pocket payments, 45% to 50%, is similar among income groups. The reason why the low income group has the same percentage out-of-pocket payments

Table 3
Mean expense per person with a visit and percent distribution of payment sources by family income, 2000

Family income	Population with visit in millions	Mean expense per visit (US dollars)	Source of payment (percent distribution)			
			Out-of-pocket	Private insurance	Medicaid	Other
Low	22.9	395	45.6	24.0	22.8	7.4
Middle	36.5	467	51.6	40.0	3.1	5.3
High	56.5	529	47.9	48.3	0.3	3.5

Data from Brown E, Manski R. Dental services: use expenses, and sources of payment, 1996–2000. Rockville (MD): Agency for Healthcare Research and Quality; 2004. MEPS Research Findings #20. AHRQ Pub. No. 04–0018.

as the other two groups is because most low income people are not covered by the Medicaid program. Usually, only people with incomes 125% of the Federal Poverty Level or lower are eligible, and even then most states only cover children. When adults are covered, the benefits are usually very limited.

As expected, private insurance coverage is mainly seen in the higher income group. Interestingly, 24% of low income families are enrolled in private dental insurance plans. These people account for a large percentage of the low income population that does visit a dentist each year.

Medicaid is almost entirely limited to the low income population, but even within this group only 22.8% are covered by this public dental insurance plan for the poor. The other payment source consists mainly of government programs for special populations such as veterans and HIV/AIDS patients.

Fig. 3 compares Medicaid expenditures for dentist and physician services in 1980 to 2005 [5]. The Medicaid program was enacted in 1965, and in 1970 there was relatively little difference between payments to dentists and physicians. Starting in 1990, payments to physicians increased dramatically, whereas payments to dentists rose more slowly. Considering that enrollment in the Medicaid dental program increased over this 35-year time period, actual per eligible payments grew very slowly [16].

Policy implications

Access disparities in the United States are mainly the result of inadequate public dental insurance for low income families. In most states, Medicaid offers limited benefits for adults, if any, and Medicaid reimbursement fees are

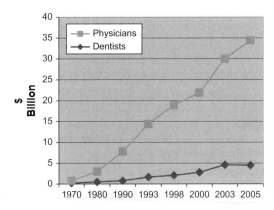

Fig. 3. Medicaid payments to dentists and physicians, 1980 to 2005. (*Data from* Center for Medicare and Medicaid Services. National health expenditures aggregate amounts and average annual percent change, by type of expenditure: selected calendar years 1960–2005. Available at: http://www.cms.hhs.gov/NationalHealthExpendData/downloads/tables.pdf. Accessed July 2007.)

so low that only 26% of dentists nationally see Medicaid patients [17]. These limitations are the primary reason why use by low income populations is so low.

Many low income areas have few dentists as demonstrated by the large number of dental health professional shortage areas. In large part, this is because dentists cannot make an adequate living practicing in these areas. If Medicaid paid competitive fees, over the long run, an adequate number of dentists would eventually move into these shortage areas to serve the population, or existing dentists would take on more Medicaid patients. An example supporting this statement comes from the state of Michigan [18]. In 52 counties, the Medicaid plan for children was turned over to a private insurer that paid the same fees as privately insured children and administered the Medicaid plan the same as the private plan. Without any increase in the number of area dentists, Medicaid use increased from about 35% to 55%. The latter is the same use rate seen in privately insured children from middle income families.

Interestingly, access to medical care for children enrolled in the Medicaid program is as high, or higher, than for middle income children [19] because the fees paid to physicians and hospitals for treating Medicaid eligible children are closer to competitive private sector fees when compared with dental fees. Also, safety net clinics that provide medical care to low income children are much more extensive than dental clinics. This observation clearly suggests that dental care access disparities for low income children could be reduced substantially if Medicaid dental fees were more competitive, and if most safety net medical clinics provided dental services.

Unfortunately, many health planners still view the dental disparities problem in terms of the population-to-dentist ratio. These people call for large increases in the number of dental graduates, assuming that more dentists will increase competition and lower the rate of increase in dental fees. Although more dentists will slow the rate of fee increases, this will mainly benefit middle and upper income families. Most low income families still will not have the resources to purchase private sector dental services.

A final issue is the reason why Medicaid dental fees are so much lower relative to private sector fees when compared with fees for physician and hospital services. At one level, this allocation of resources to public dental benefits reflects larger societal views of the value of different health care services. Unfortunately, dental (and mental health services) receive relatively low priority.

A second reason is the lobbying power of other health care professions and organizations dealing with state legislatures. In most states, the state hospital association spends millions of dollars trying to convince legislators that hospitals should receive full payment (ie, comparable to private sector fees) for treating Medicaid patients. They are not completely successful in this effort, but hospitals fees are often in the 70th to 80th percentile of private sector fees. In contrast, state dental associations spend much less on lobbying legislatures. The different health care occupations and organizations are in competition to get a bigger share of Medicaid funds, and dentists do not generally fair well in this competition. It is no surprise that Medicaid dental fees are very low in most states. There is no simple way to overcome these two barriers to more competitive Medicaid dental fees.

Reasons for increased dental expenditures

Since 1980, dental expenditures have risen an average of 7.2% per year, almost twice the rate of increase in the consumer price index. The key question is what accounts for this high rate of increase in dental expenditures. Three potential reasons include population growth, inflation in dental fees, and increased use.

Population growth

From 1980 to 2005, the US population increased from 230 million to 297 million people. With 67 million more people in 2005, it is obvious that more people will seek dental care. As seen in Table 4, population growth accounts for one percentage point of the average annual growth of 7.2% in dental expenditures.

Fees

The fees that dentists charge for their services could also account for some of the increase in expenditures. Fig. 4 compares the increase in the dental price index and the consumer price index. For the period from 1980 to 2005, the first index measures the price level of dental services and the second index the price level for all goods and services. Over 25 years, the dental price index rose from 78.9 to 324.0 (5.5% per year) and the consumer price index from 82.3 to 297.0 (3.2% per year); therefore, dental fee inflation increased 2.3% per year. In total, general inflation and dental fee inflation account for 76% of the 7.2% increase in dental expenditures (see Table 4). This level of fee inflation suggests a tightening in the supply of dental services relative to the demand for care.

Table 4
Contributions of increases in population, fee inflation, and per capita use to the average annual increase (7.2%) in dental expenditures, 1980 to 2005

Factor	Percentage point contribution
Population	1.0
Dental price index	5.5[a]
Use	0.7
Total	7.2

[a] The consumer price index is 3.2%.

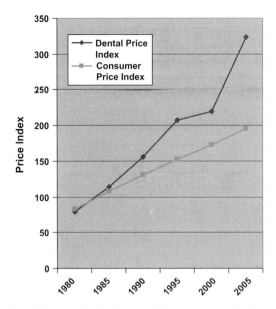

Fig. 4. Comparison of the dental price index and the consumer price index, 1980 to 2005.

Utilization

Another possibility is growth in the per capita use of dental services, that is, people may be going to dentists more often, and when they do go, they may receive a more expensive mix of services. Fig. 5 presents per capita expenditures for dental care, adjusting for fee inflation from 1980 to 2005. It is clear that per capita use has increased in inflation adjusted (or real) dollars from $73.41 per person to $90.03 per person, a 36% increase in 25 years. This analysis cannot differentiate how much of this change is due to a greater number of visits per person versus a more expensive mix of services for those receiving care. Because data from other studies indicate that per capita use has remained relatively steady [3], the increase is probably mainly the result of a more expensive mix of services, such as composites for amalgams and

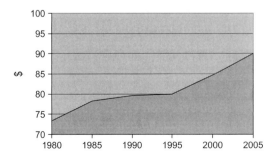

Fig. 5. Per capita expenditures for dental care adjusted for inflation in dental fees, 1980 to 2005.

implants for missing teeth. As indicated in Table 4, increased use accounts for 0.7 percentage points of the average 7.2% increase in annual dental expenditures.

Summary

Based on the evidence available, what predictions can be made about the future financing of dental care? In terms of access to care, the future looks bright for middle and upper income families that have the resources to purchase dental services in the private sector using a combination of private dental insurance and out-of-pocket payments. Even though the oral health of the population has improved over the past 25 years [20], the demand for dental care continues to increase. There are several reasons for this increased demand.

- Young children below the age of 5 years and the elderly, two groups that traditionally have been low users of dental care, are going to the dentist more often [20].
- Many people in good oral health are willing to spend significant amounts of money to maintain their dentitions.
- New preventive, diagnostic, and treatment technologies are becoming available that are more effective but also more expensive than the technologies they replaced.
- The number of people with private dental insurance has remained steady for the past 5 years, even though enrollment in private medical insurance has declined.

All of these factors suggest that the demand for care will continue to increase. Indeed, this conclusion is supported by federal government projections that dental care expenditures will continue to grow close to current rates for at least the next 7 years.

Although overall use is likely to increase for the foreseeable future, the wide disparities in access to dental care may well persist. Low income populations will continue to have major problems accessing dental care. There is little indication that federal and state governments are willing to increase Medicaid dental fees to competitive levels, to expand Medicaid enrollment to include low income adults, or to provide enrolled adults with a more comprehensive set of dental benefits.

As long as medical care costs continue to increase much faster than the general economy, public payers will be hard pressed to find more funds to cover dental care. Furthermore, as previously noted, other health care providers will do their best to lobby government to allocate any new monies to their areas of concern. The demand for increasing payments to hospitals, physicians, pharmacies, and long-term care facilities is certain to continue, and it will be difficult for dentistry to compete with these other groups for a greater share of Medicaid funds.

There is some discussion of a major reorganization of the health care financing system. In fact, several states have proposed new financing schemes that will decrease the number of uninsured [21]. Unfortunately, these plans have not given serious attention to the problem of controlling health care costs. Until this is done, it is unlikely that efforts to just increase enrollment will be successful in the long run.

In terms of dentists' incomes, Fig. 6 shows the increase in the average income of full-time general dentists and specialists over the past 15 years [22]. As is well known to most dentists, this has been a period of rapidly growing incomes. For the first time in the United States, the average general dentist now earns considerably more than the average general medical practitioner. The question is how long this trend will continue.

The two primary factors that will drive dentists' incomes are the demand for care and the supply of services. The demand for dental services has already been discussed and appears promising. The supply of dental services is another matter and has not been discussed herein. The significant inflation in dental fees strongly suggests that the demand for services has been greater than the supply for the past 10 to 15 years. Obviously, if there is a significant increase in the supply of services and the supply exceeds the demand, the incomes of dentists will grow at a slower rate.

The supply of services could increase for several reasons. The first reason is an increase in the number of dentists. For the past 15 years, the dentist-to-population ratio has been decreasing as the result of the closure of seven dental schools and class size reductions at many others from 1975 to 1985. This era is coming to an end [22]. At least five new dental schools have started or will start in the next few years, and it is likely that several more will be established. Interestingly, most of these new institutions are associated with schools of osteopathic medicine. These private schools tend to

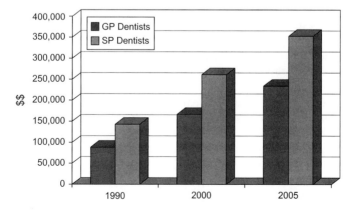

Fig. 6. Income of full-time general dentists and specialists, 1990 to 2005. (*From* Bailit H, Beazoglou T, Formicola A, et al. US state-supported dental schools: financial projections and implications. J Dent Educ 2006;70(3):251; with permission.)

have large classes and charge high tuition. Furthermore, many established schools have started 2-year programs to give international dental graduates US dental degrees. In aggregate, the new schools and the international dental student programs are expected to increase the number of dental graduates from 10% to 20% within the next 10 years. This means another 500 to 1000 graduates per year.

Another factor that will increase the supply of services is the expansion of roles of dental paraprofessionals. In this regard, the use of dental therapists by an Alaskan native organization is a major new development. Therapists provide restorative care to children and adults and work under the indirect supervision of dentists. A training program for therapists is now being established at the University of Washington, and therapists may soon be operating in tribal dental clinics throughout the country (Dr. Peter Milgrom, personal communication, 2007). In some states, they may eventually provide care in federally and state funded dental clinics outside of tribal areas. Longer term, some states may allow therapists to be employed in private dental offices. This practice is now accepted in Australia, the United Kingdom, some Canadian provinces, and New Zealand. Clearly, therapists will increase the supply of dental services.

The expansion of the duties and the greater use of traditional allied dental health providers are also increasing. Dentists are employing more assistants, hygienists, and administrative staff, and many states are expanding the roles of assistants and hygienists. Studies suggest that the greater use of allied dental health staff makes dentists more productive; they are able to provide more services per unit time which is, in effect, an increase in the supply of services [23,24].

It appears that the supply of dental services will increase substantially in the next 10 years with more dental school graduates, a new midlevel practitioner, and greater use of allied dental health personnel. Whether this supply increase will grow faster than the increase in demand for care is an open question. If it does, this will lead to less inflation in dental fees and slower growth of dentists' incomes.

The most important point is that the changes in the financing of dental care have major implications for the oral health of the American people and the incomes of practicing dentists. Both dental organizations and dentists need to pay careful attention to any proposed changes in the financing of dental care and take an active role in influencing legislation.

References

[1] Catlin A, Cowan C, Heffler S, et al. National health spending in 2005: the slowdown continues. Health Aff 2007;26(1):142–53.
[2] Widstrom E, Eaton K. Oral health care systems in the extended European Union. Oral Health Prev Dent 2004;3:155–94.

[3] Brown E, Manski R. Dental services: use expenses, and sources of payment, 1996–2000. Rockville (MD): Agency for Healthcare Research and Quality; 2004. MEPS Research Findings #20. AHRQ Pub. No. 04–0018.

[4] Manski R, Macek M, Moeller J. Private dental coverage: who has it and how does it influence dental visits and expenditures? J Am Dent Assoc 2002;133(11):1551–9.

[5] Center for Medicare and Medicaid Services. National health expenditures aggregate amounts and average annual percent change, by type of expenditure: selected calendar years 1960–2005. Available at: http://www.cms.hhs.gov/NationalHealthExpendData/downloads/tables.pdf. Accessed July 2007.

[6] American Heart Association. 2007 update: economic costs of cardiovascular diseases. Heart Diseases and Stroke Statistics 2007:37.

[7] Meropol N, Schulman K. Cost of cancer care: issues and implications. J Clin Oncol 2007; 25(2):180–6.

[8] Heffler S, Smith S, Keehan S, et al. Health spending projections through 2013. Health Affairs (Web Exclusive) February 11, 2004.

[9] Bailit HL. Dental insurance, managed care and traditional practice. J Am Dent Assoc 1999; 130:1721–7.

[10] Dubay L, Holahan J, Cook A. The uninsured and the affordability of health insurance coverage. Health Affairs 2007;26(1):22–30.

[11] Cohen L. Opportunities for international research collaborations: mechanisms for advancement. J Dent Educ 1999;63(3):263–227.

[12] Gilbert G, Duncan R, Heft M, et al. Dental health attitudes among dentate black and white adults. Med Care 1997;35(3):255–71.

[13] Smithwick K. Companies modifying plan designs, but avoiding cost shifting. Managed Dental Care 2005;10(7):1, 5–6.

[14] US Department of Labor. Bureau of Labor Statistics, percent of all workers participating in dental care benefits, all private industry, 1999–2006. Available at: http://data.bls.gov/PDQ/servlet/SurveyOutputServlet. Accessed July 2007.

[15] Claxton G, Gabel J, Gil I, et al. Health benefits in 2006: premium increases moderate, enrollment in consumer-directed health plans remains modest. Health Affairs Web Exclusive 2007; 26(5):1407–16.

[16] Center for Medicare and Medicaid Services. Table 88. Number of Medicaid persons served (beneficiaries) by eligibility group: fiscal years 1975–2002. Available at: http://www.cms.hhs.gov/MedicareMedicaidStatSupp/LT/itemdetail.asp?filterType=none&filterByDID=-99&sortByDID=1&sortOrder=ascending&itemID=CMS060512&intNumPerPage=10. Accessed July 2007.

[17] American Dental Association. Dentist's participation in Medicaid programs: 2000 survey of current issues in dentistry. American Dental Association 2001:1–10.

[18] Eklund S, Pittman J, Clark S. Michigan Medicaid's Healthy Kids dental program: an assessment of the first 12 months. J Am Dent Assoc 2003;134(11):1509–15.

[19] Wobus D, Olin G. Health care expenses: poor, near poor, and low income people in the United States civilian noninstitutionalized population, 2002. Agency for Healthcare Research and Quality. Working Paper No. 05016, July 2005.

[20] Dye B, Smith T, Lewis B, et al. Trends in oral health status: United States, 1988–1994 and 1999–2004. National Center for Health Statistics. Vital Health Stat 2007;11(248):1–92.

[21] Holahan J, Blumberg L. Massachusetts health care reform: a look at the issues. Health Affairs 2006;25:W432–46.

[22] Bailit H, Beazoglou T, Formicola A, et al. US state-supported dental schools: financial projections and implications. J Dent Educ 2006;70(3):246–57.

[23] Beazoglou T, Heffley D, Brown LJ, et al. The importance of productivity in estimating need for dentists. J Am Dent Assoc 2002;133:1399–404.

[24] Wang N. Productivity in dental care for children: factors influencing the time spent delivering dental care. Community Dent Health 1994;11(4):227–32.

ELSEVIER
SAUNDERS

THE DENTAL
CLINICS
OF NORTH AMERICA

Dent Clin N Am 52 (2008) 297–318

Oral Health Disparities
in the United States

Amit Chattopadhyay,
PhD, MPH, MDS, BDS (Hons)[a,b,*]

[a]*Department of Epidemiology, University of Kentucky College of Public Health,
Room # 209-C, 121 Washington Avenue, Lexington, KY 40536, USA*
[b]*Division of Dental Public Health, Department of Oral Health Sciences,
University of Kentucky College of Dentistry, Lexington, KY, USA*

Research into health disparities has grown tremendously since welfare economic studies associating poverty and health outcomes gained worldwide recognition: "... the poor should not be regarded as an undifferentiated mass, but that one should rather identify particular groups which have been struck by a catastrophic imbalance between needs and resources. Smallholders, farm laborers, tenant farmers and herdsmen may well all be poor, but the ways in which they are affected by famine can differ greatly" [1,2].

Essentially, disparity is the occurrence of differences between any two or more groups. As a dispassionate term, it is devoid of any qualifications and denotes existence of differences. However, health or social awareness and activism impart a qualification to health disparities, underlining a need to change status quo and remove disparities to improve health of those whose health status lies below that of the chosen reference. The National Institutes of Health has defined disparities as the "differences in the incidence, prevalence, mortality, and burden of diseases and other adverse health conditions that exist among specific population groups in the United States" [3]. Other entities, such as the National Cancer Institute [4] and Minority Health and Health Disparities Research and Education Act of 2000 [5], have defined disparities slightly differently, although the major focus is on the existence of differences between groups.

In the United States, disparities have been observed in oral health outcomes by gender, race or ethnicity, education, income, disability, geographic

* Department of Epidemiology, University of Kentucky College of Public Health, Room # 209-C, 121 Washington Avenue, Lexington, KY 40536.

E-mail address: achat4@email.uky.edu

0011-8532/08/$ - see front matter © 2008 Elsevier Inc. All rights reserved.
doi:10.1016/j.cden.2007.11.001

location, and sexual orientation [6]. The National Institute for Dental and Craniofacial Research (NIDCR) has set up a Health Disparities Research Program, with "a plan to eliminate craniofacial, oral and dental health disparities," in response to the growing awareness that despite improvements in some oral health status indicators, the burden of disease is not evenly distributed across all segments of societies [7].

Equality, equity, and disparity

Oral health equality implies the existence of equal oral health attributes among different groups, whereas the term "equity" incorporates an ethical quality to equality or disparity. Therefore, when we state, for example, that the burden of periodontal disease is greater in non-Hispanic Blacks, compared with non-Hispanic Whites [6], we just make a statement about existent disparity. However, when we make an ethical qualification stating that the above disparity is unacceptable and should be eliminated or reduced, then we choose to a stand in favor of oral health equity. Merely documenting oral health disparity in the absence of oral health equity does not allow us to take considered action toward the betterment of population oral health status.

As identified by NIDCR, disadvantaged and underserved population subgroups that fit within the research activities supported by the Health Disparities Research Program to eliminate or reduce disparity [7] include:

All race and ethnic populations with health disparities, including African American, Hispanic (Mexican, Puerto Rican, Cuban, Central or South American, or other Spanish culture or origin, regardless of race), American Indian or Alaskan Native, and Asian or Pacific Islanders;
Low income rural (eg, Appalachian) or urban dwellers;
Special needs populations (eg, physically or mentally disabled);
People living with HIV/AIDS;
The elderly; and
Home-bound and institutionalized individuals

Existing oral health disparities

The first ever report on oral health, by the Surgeon General of the United States in the year 2000, brought into focus the profound oral health disparities existing in the country [6]. Not only are there profound differences in the population in accessing the oral health care delivery system, but it has also been shown that even after accessing this system, there are substantial differences in clinical condition, awareness of treatment options, treatment discussions, treatment recommendations, and treatment received by different social groups [8–12].

Disparities in oral health status

Dental caries

Despite remarkable reduction in the prevalence of dental caries in the United States, childhood dental caries are still highly prevalent among the socially disadvantaged (racial or ethnic minority, poor, rural, immigrants) sections of United States society. According to the National Health and Nutrition Examination Survey (NHANES), caries experience in primary teeth in children aged 2 to 5 years has increased from the periods of 1988–2004 (NHANES III), to 1999–2004 (NHANES 1999–2004) [13]. Although the overall prevalence of dental caries status of permanent teeth has decreased over the last 15 years (since the 1988–1994 NHANES III survey), profound disparities in disease prevalence, treatment received, and treatment outcomes continue to remain between various social groups [14].

Sequelae of dental caries (such as pain and complex dental treatment needs), therefore, also are more prevalent among children from these socially disadvantaged groups [15]. Children from these groups experience the greatest amount of oral disease, the most extensive disease, and the most frequent use of dental services for pain relief [6,16].

Dental diseases in early childhood impact the growth, function, behavior, and comfort of the affected children. The twin disparities of poor oral health and lack of dental care are most evident among low-income preschool children, who are twice as likely to have cavities as are higher income children [16]. These disparities continue into adolescence and young adulthood, although to a lesser degree. Disparities in oral health status and access to dental care are also evident when comparing African American, Hispanic, and Native American children to Caucasian children, and when comparing children of parents with low educational attainment to children of parents with higher educational attainment. The fastest growing populations of children are those that currently have the highest disease rates and the lowest amount of dental care [16].

Tooth loss

Race and socio-economic disadvantage are strong determinants of tooth loss [10]. Cunha-Cruz and colleagues [17] examined whether socio-economic disparities in edentulism had changed over time, by investigating the socio-economic disparities in edentulism between 1972 and 2001 using NHANES data for those years. They reported that overall, prevalence of edentulism remained approximately stable over the three decades, being 10.6% in 1972, 12.1% in 1991, and 11.3% in 2001. Furthermore, although the absolute difference in prevalence of edentulism between low and high socio-economic position groups remained unchanged, disparity was substantial for those who did not visit a dentist in the previous year when compared with those who did [17].

The Florida dental care study found that tooth loss was associated with certain practice characteristics, such as the racial mix of the practice's patient population [18]. This study reported that persons who attended practices with higher percentages of African Americans were more likely to receive a dental extraction, regardless of the individual patient's race or ethnicity. These effects remained even after adjusting for several other factors [18].

Periodontal disease

Disparities in periodontal health status in the United States follows the similar general description in that those with lower socio-economic position and minorities tend to have more and more advanced disease burden than the rest [6]. Progression of periodontal disease may be a function of several factors, including the disease status at the initial stages and factors that determine ability to use the oral health care delivery system.

A study of 53 Asian, 69 African, and 62 Hispanic Americans assessing periodontal disease progression found that the rate of attachment loss for the entire population was 0.24 mm per year, but did not find any differences among the three ethnic or racial groups. Although in bivariate analyses the study reported greater progression of disease for several factors (older study participants, professionally unskilled personnel, men, mean whole-mouth plaque, erythema, bleeding upon probing, suppuration, attachment loss, and probing depth), most of these associations disappeared on multivariable analyses to develop a final logistic regression model [19].

It is possible that observed disparities in periodontal diseases [6] are the products of more complex interaction of two or more factors. Extracting such information hidden in data might require clear hypothesis testing and well thought-out study designs that have adequate statistical power to detect the differences hypothesized. In another study with a somewhat larger sample size (232 non-Hispanic Blacks and 199 Whites), subjects from a disproportionate probability sample of community-dwelling adults were interviewed regarding demographic, psychosocial and enabling factors, dental health-related behaviors, and other risk factors, and had a comprehensive in-home dental examinations [20]. This study reported that prevalence of established periodontitis was greater among non-Hispanic Blacks (29.8%) than Whites (17.7%), with non-Hispanic Blacks having almost double the risk of established periodontitis than Whites (crude odds ratio or OR: 1.98; 95% confidence index or CI 1.43, 9.24). However, this study also reported an effect-modification of this association by dental check-up visit frequency [20]. Blacks with dental check-ups at least once a year had almost a fourfold higher odds of established periodontitis (OR 3.64; CI 1.43, 9.24), compared with Whites with similar check-up experience, whereas Blacks with a dental check-up once every 2 years or less often were more than four-fold less likely to have established periodontitis (OR 0.22; CI 0.08, 0.59) than their White counterparts in the referent group.

It has also been reported that periodontal treatment needs vary with socio-economic position, and that although most American adults need some type of periodontal treatment, these are usually within the clinical skill range of dental hygienists [21]. However, the proportion of need for complex periodontal treatment among those with lower socio-economic position is disproportionately higher than the rest. Assessing NHANES III data of 11,339 persons aged 20 to 79, Dye and Vargas [21] estimated that overall, 3% of the adult United States population required complex periodontal treatment, 90% needed scaling and prophylaxis, and nearly 5% did not need periodontal treatment or oral hygiene instruction. Using multiple logistic regression analysis, the investigators were able to report that being older, male, non-Hispanic Black (OR 2.51; CI 1.98, 3.18), having lower education or no high school (OR 2.10; CI 1.60, 2.77), smoking (current smoker, OR 2.02; CI 1.76, 2.33), or not having had a dental visit in the past year increased the likelihood of needing more complex periodontal treatment.

Oral cancer

The oral cancer story mimics that of other oral disease: despite overall decreases in oral cancer incidence and mortality rates, the disparities associated with socially disadvantaged groups have continued to exist. From 1975 through 2004, age-adjusted incidence rates (Fig. 1), age adjusted mortality rates (Fig. 2), and survival rates (Fig. 3) from oral and pharyngeal cancers are higher for men than women, being highest for Black men.

These figures suggest that overall, the Black–White disparity in oral and pharyngeal cancer can be broken into three parts.

1. Roughly similar incidence rates for Black and White women, being generally stable over the years, albeit occasional fluctuations for Black women in incidence. However, the survival and mortality rates have consistently been in favor of White women compared with Black women.
2. Substantial and prolonged disparity in incidence rates between Black and White men, which seem to have found a meeting point in the early 2000s. Incidence rates in Black men seem to have started to decline steadily from the mid 1980s, and current data suggests that the disparity with White men in age-adjusted incidence has been eliminated. However, age adjusted mortality rates and survival rates tell a very different story, with substantial disparities in favor of White men.
3. Despite changes, the disparities in incidence, mortality, and survival between men and women, in favor of women, has remained approximately steady over the years.

A recent study reported that age adjusted mortality rates were 82% higher for Black men compared with White men, but rates were similar for Black and White women. Five-year relative survival rates for patients diagnosed during the period 1995 to 2001 were higher for Whites than for Blacks and lowest for Black males [22]. Interestingly, the survival rates of oral cancer have remained fairly stable over the decades. Similar results have been reported from Florida [23], Kentucky [24], North Carolina [25], and elsewhere.

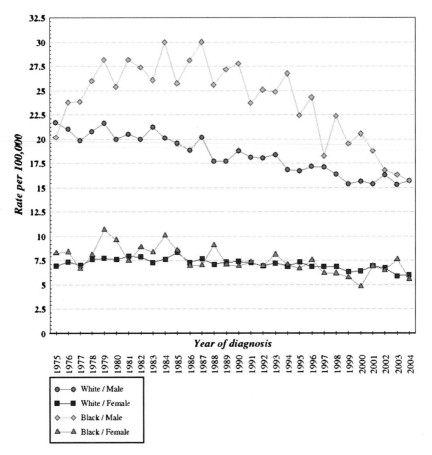

Fig. 1. Age adjusted incidence by race and sex for oral and pharyngeal cancer. (*Data from* Surveillance, Epidemiology, and End Results (SEER) Program (www.seer.cancer.gov.) SEER*-Stat Database: Incidence - SEER 9 Regs Limited-Use, Nov 2006 Sub (1973–2004), National Cancer Institute, DCCPS, Surveillance Research Program, Cancer Statistics Branch, released April 2007, based on the November 2006 submission.)

Table 1 shows the stages of oral and pharyngeal cancer at presentation from the Surveillance Epidemiology and End Results (SEER) data in 5-year groups every 10-years. Whereas the overall trends are similar for Blacks and Whites, the greater proportion of earlier stage presentation among Whites over Blacks stands out. Although the proportion of regional spread presentations increased for all, the proportion of increase is greater for White men compared with Black men (10% versus 18%, respectively) from 1985–1989 to 1996–2003.

Orofacial pain

The Florida dental study, using standardized telephonic surveys assessing 724 dentate adults above 45 years of age, has contributed substantially

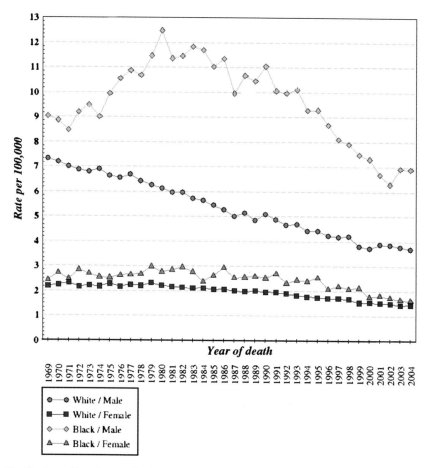

Fig. 2. Age adjusted mortality by race or sex for oral and pharyngeal cancer. (*Data from* Surveillance, Epidemiology, and End Results (SEER) Program (www.seer.cancer.gov) SEER*-Stat Database: Mortality - All COD, Public-Use With State, Total United States (1969–2004), National Cancer Institute, DCCPS, Surveillance Research Program, Cancer Statistics Branch, released April 2007. Underlying mortality data provided by NCHS at www.cdc.gov/nchs.)

toward understanding prevailing disparities in self-reported orofacial pain in the United States [26]. This study reported that lower socio-economic position was associated with greater self-reported pain and pain impact at many orofacial sites. This observation suggests that persons with lower socio-economic position are at increased risk for orofacial pain and pain-related behavioral impact, measured as pain having reduced their daily activities or motivating them to take some action in response to it. Furthermore, this association of socio-economic position and orofacial pain varied by sex: only men with lower financial status were at increased risk for orofacial pain-related behavioral impact in at least one site [26]. However, in a study of senior citizens (65 years or older), although prevalence of self-reported

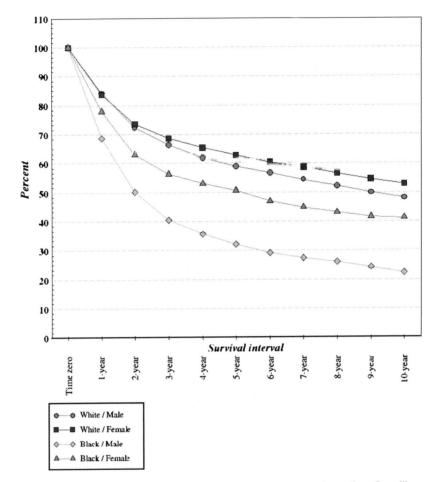

Fig. 3. Survival from oral and pharyngeal cancer by race or sex. (*Data from* Surveillance, Epidemiology, and End Results (SEER) Program (www.seer.cancer.gov.) SEER*Stat Database: Incidence - SEER 17 Regs Limited-Use, Nov 2006 Sub (1973–2004 varying), National Cancer Institute, DCCPS, Surveillance Research Program, Cancer Statistics Branch, released April 2007, based on the November 2006 submission.)

orofacial pain did not differ by race or ethnicity, there were differences in behavioral impact associated with pain [27]. This latter study found that Blacks reported greater behavioral impact, even after adjusting for socio-economic status, approach to health care, and intensity of pain.

Persons with special care needs

Oral health related disparities are perhaps most evident and severe when persons with special care needs are assessed against those who do not need special care for management of their oral health problems. The Surgeon General's report on oral health stated that people living below the poverty

Table 1

SEER Stage distribution by race and sex for oral cavity and pharynx cancer, all ages, SEER 9 registries for 1975–1979, 1985–1989, and 1996–2003

	White			Black		
All	1975–1979	1985–1989	1996–2003	1975–1979	1985–1989	1996 2003
Percent localized	41%	40%	36%	26%	18%	20%
Percent regional	37%	43%	50%	49%	56%	60%
Percent distant	12%	9%	9%	17%	19%	16%
Percent un-staged	10%	8%	5%	8%	7%	4%
	White men			Black men		
Men	1975–1979	1985–1989	1996–2003	1975–1979	1985–1989	1996–2003
Percent localized	41%	39%	34%	25%	15%	16%
Percent regional	37%	44%	52%	51%	57%	63%
Percent distant	12%	9%	9%	17%	22%	17%
Percent un-staged	10%	8%	4%	7%	6%	4%
	White women			Black women		
Women	1975–1979	1985–1989	1996–2003	1975–1979	1985–1989	1996–2003
Percent localized	40%	41%	42%	30%	26%	29%
Percent regional	39%	42%	43%	46%	53%	54%
Percent distant	11%	8%	8%	16%	13%	12%
Percent un-staged	9%	9%	6%	8%	8%	5%

level and those with mental retardation or physical disabilities have poorer oral health than the general population [6]. One study examined the oral health status of intellectually disabled persons, with or without a physical disability, by screening 12,099 Special Olympics athletes at 53 sites, including 1,891 people from seven states in the southeastern United States [28]. The examinations were performed by volunteer dentists and dental students. Oral health disparities in this study sample were associated with poverty. Restricting the analysis by age, the study reported that athletes from the very poor southeastern states were 1.6 times (OR 1.64; 95% CI 1.10–2.46) more likely to have restorations and almost one-third as likely (OR 0.35; 95% CI 0.21–0.60) to have sealants than were athletes from the poor states. Adults with developmental disabilities generally have a more sedentary lifestyle, poorer general health, and multiple comorbidities when compared with those without such disabilities [29]. Nursing home residents, mostly elderly persons who can barely perform or need support for activities of daily living, have poor oral health and inadequate access to oral health care. Further details are discussed in the article by Chalmers and Ettinger elsewhere in this issue.

These persons with special needs also have poorer rates of insurance coverage and have substantially lesser rates of use of the health care delivery system. These issues also translate to their poorer oral health as compared with the general population. Current oral health surveillance methods do not cover this population, although the potential of substantially elevated unmet needs among this population are perhaps the greatest.

Elderly persons

Dental caries (coronal and root caries) continue to be a problem requiring public health attention for the noninstitutionalized elderly, especially African Americans who also use the oral health care system less and have poorer insurance coverage. Those elderly persons with lower socio-economic position, living in rural areas, or those who have special care requirements, have greater unmet needs compared with the other elderly Americans. Further details are discussed in an article by Chalmers and Ettinger elsewhere in this issue.

Disparities in oral health service access

Service use

Utilization of available oral health care services is a good marker for how well the current oral health care delivery system is working. Utilization of the oral health care delivery system varies by the socio-economic position and racial or ethnic characteristic of the population. Analysis using a nationally representative sample from the 1996 Medical Expenditure Panel Survey demonstrated that there was an approximate twofold difference in the proportion of persons accessing the oral health care delivery system between the lowest income group (28.1% for persons below 200% of the federal poverty line) and the highest income group (55.8% for persons above 400% of the federal poverty line) [30]. Other findings from the study include: Non-Hispanic Blacks and Hispanics were less likely to access the system than Whites or other race and ethnic groups; men were less likely to access the system than women; and people not in employment were less likely to access the system than those employed [30].

Assessing the recent expansions in Medicaid and the State Children's Health Insurance Program (SCHIP), a recent study reported that overall, use of ambulatory dental care has increased dramatically for children over the past two decades [31]. In 1983, more than one in three children (38.5%) had no dental care within the previous 12 months, which decreased to 26.3% in 2001. However, frequency of unmet dental care did not change from 1997–1998 to 2001–2002. The same study did not find any changes in income disparities for unmet dental needs [31]. Even today, as earlier, low income children are less likely to visit the dentist in part because of their family's competing needs for limited resources, shortage of pediatric dentists, and dentists not taking uninsured or publicly insured patients [15].

Over the past decade, the proportion of the American population reporting to have visited a dentist in the previous year has remained fairly constant (ie, 69% in 1996, 68% in 1999, 69.5% in 2002, and 69% in 2004) [6,32,33]. A New York State survey among minorities found that self-reported visits to a dentist in the previous year was only 63% [30], 10% lower than the estimated state average. Perhaps it would be safe to assume that these proportions of differences would be substantially higher if undocumented immigrants were accounted for. Therefore, unless some type of immigration reform occurs to bring undocumented immigrants into the legal system with impunity, disparities for this group will continue to be high and perhaps increasing, compared with the rest of the United States population.

Substantial disparities exist in the use of orthodontic services among high school students [34]. This study reported that the odds of being orthodontically treated were 8.7 times greater among those with dental visits within the past year than among those without, and three times greater among Caucasians than among other ethnic groups. Furthermore, ethnic minority groups had 2.6 greater odds of needing orthodontic treatment than Caucasians [34].

In the adjusted regression models, Black patients and those with unknown race were less likely overall to receive root canal therapy than Whites, whereas Asians were more likely. Among patients with eligibility for continuing and comprehensive dental care, Blacks were less likely and Asians more likely to receive root canals than Whites. For patients covered only for emergency dental care, Hispanics had a higher likelihood of receiving root canal therapy. Among all other types of coverage, there were no significant racial differences in the care received [35].

Household income plays a major role in a family's ability to access the oral health care system. It is well established that adults and children from poor households have the most oral health disease and access the system the least. Paradoxically, children in poverty—those living in households with annual gross incomes under $16,500 for a family of four—or near poverty (those in family households with incomes between $16,500 and $33,000), also have the highest rates of dental insurance coverage, primarily through Medicaid programs and SCHIP [16]. Medicaid-eligible children who have cavities have twice the numbers of decayed teeth and twice the number of visits for pain relief, but fewer total dental visits, compared with children coming from families with higher incomes. Fewer preventive visits for services such as sealants increase the burden of disease in low-income children [16].

Geographic and neighborhood issues

In addition to existing statistical techniques, recent advances in Geographic Intelligent Systems (GIS) software applications have allowed investigators to assess geographic disparities in an easily understandable format, which includes graphic analysis, overlays, and much more. These methods allow a readily appreciable pictorial description of differences of attributes between geographic zones. In conjunction with existing methods, GIS applications strengthen program planning and visual interpretation of information. For example, individual and overlay maps were produced in a study to examine the geographic distribution of New York City adults aged 65 and older, by race or ethnicity and poverty status [36]. This study found that Black race, Hispanic ethnicity, and poverty status tended to occur together geo-spatially among elders in Northern Manhattan and the South Bronx, information that can be incorporated in planning oral health service delivery for elders [36].

Oral health disparities exist among United States adults living in rural and urban areas. Using NHANES III data, Vargas and colleagues [37] reported that compared with urban residents, rural residents were less likely to report a dental visit in the past year and were more likely to be edentulous. Adults living in rural areas were more likely to report having unmet dental care needs and were less likely to have had a dental visit in the past year, compared with adults living in urban areas [37]. The prevalence of edentulism among rural adults was 16.3%, almost twice that of urban adults. Caries experience also was more likely to be greater among adults residing in rural areas.

A study in Harlem, New York reported that those with low income, unemployed, and uninsured, had poorer oral health status, emphasizing that the privately insured were almost twice as likely to have seen a dentist for oral health problems as were the uninsured [38]. Inability to pay for dental services received (unpaid care) may be a marker for low socio-economic position, and may be adopted as a possible coping strategy for obtaining minimal, but essential services when in need. Data from the 1996 Medical Expenditure Panel Survey suggests that unpaid care was higher for those living in northeast and in west census tract zones when compared with other areas, and for the oldest age groups, women, low income, unemployed, Hispanics, those with Medicaid, and those undergoing more than one dental procedure type [39]. The differences in unpaid care between geographic areas (census tracts zones) persisted even after adjustment for other important variables. Although it may not be easy to explain such differences, ecologic comparison of evidences from other studies may suggest the possibility of some association with the distribution of undocumented laborers who generally live in an "informal-economy." These individuals may resist accessing the oral health care delivery system out of fear of possible backlash from other sections of the political system, to avoid being discovered and deported. Such possibilities are becoming important for the American health care delivery system, as the system tries ways to provide health care to this vulnerable population.

Neighborhoods may impart unique qualities to oral health status of residents beyond socio-economic position and individual risk factors. An assessment of the relationship between neighborhood effects and the severity of dental caries among low-income African Americans using multi-level methods suggested there is significant variation in the severity of caries between low-income neighborhood clusters [40]. This study demonstrated that caries severity was lower in areas with a higher number of churches, whereas it was greater in areas with a higher number of grocery stores in the clusters, after accounting for several individual characteristics. Only 14% of the interindividual variability in dental caries in this study was explained by classic individual risk factors [40].

More remote areas of the United States also exhibit profound between-region disparities in oral health. For example, a disproportionately higher proportion of American Indian and Alaska Native children have oral disease, compared with the general population of American children, apart from having limited access to professional oral health care [41]. It is well documented that the Indian Health Service and American Indian and Alaska Native tribal leaders face a significant problem in ensuring care for the oral health of these populations [41].

Table 2 lists the national oral health attributes from the 2004 Behavioral Risk Factor Surveillance System (BRFSS) and those of the states that reported state-wide surveys to the National Oral Health Surveillance System (NOHSS). The NOHSS is a collaborative effort between the Centers for Disease Control Division of Oral Health and the Association of State and Territorial Dental Directors that was established in 2001. NOHSS is designed to monitor the burden of oral disease, use of the oral health care delivery system, and the status of community water fluoridation on both a national and state level. NOHSS includes eight indicators of oral health, information on state dental programs, and links to other important sources of oral health information.

There exist profound disparities between states in almost all measured oral health indicators. For example, Connecticut ranks on the top for the proportion of persons who reported having visited a dentist in the previous year (79.3%), whereas Mississippi ranks at the bottom (58%), being 21 percentage points lower than Connecticut and 11 percentage points below the national average (69%). Connecticut ranked on the top for the proportion of persons reporting having their teeth cleaned in the previous year (79.1%). Mississippi was at the bottom (56.6%); only the Virgin Islands were lower than Mississippi (55.4%). Similarly, substantial between-state disparities exist for other oral health indicators. At the state level, the average household income of the state seemed to correlate well with the state's oral health indicators and national ranking (see Table 2).

Provision of services

Different clinicians interpret clinical data quite differently, and their advice may vary in the absence of practice guidelines. Their interpretations and resulting actions may define patterns unique to their practices and the areas these practices serve. Therefore, dental practice patterns may contribute to existing disparities and their propagation [9]. A recent study examining this issue in periodontal decision making found that experienced practitioners showed most variation, and noted that clinicians linked to a training center shared a common treatment philosophy more often than those outside such centers [12]. This shared philosophy, however, varied

Table 2

Oral health indicators [% (95% CI)] reported to the National Oral Health Surveillance System exhibits disparities between states (and from national average) for all available oral health indicators

2004 BRFSS	Dental visit	Teeth cleaning	All teeth lost	Six or more teeth lost	Sealants	Caries	Untreated caries
National Average	69.0	69.0	20.5	45.9	—	—	—
Alabama	67.2	69.3	31.9	56.3	—	—	—
Alaska	68.3	64.4	23.0	50.9	52.5 (49.5–55.3)	65.2 (62.7–67.8)	28.1 (25.5–30.7)
Arizona	66.6	65.9	15.0	36.7	36.2 (31.4–41.1)	66.7 (63.2–70.2)	39.4 (34.9–44.0)
Arkansas	59.7	57.7	24.7	53.8	24.5 (21.3–27.5)	72.3 (68.9–75.5)	42.2 (38.4–45.8)
California	68.7	67.9	13.8	36.3	27.6 (25.7–29.4)	70.9 (69.1–72.8)	28.7 (27.0–30.4)
Colorado	71.1	69.6	18.1	41.2	35.2 (30.1–40.2)	57.2 (52.5–61.9)	26.1 (22.1–30.0)
Connecticut	79.3	79.1	12.4	38.3	—	—	—
Delaware	76.4	77.8	21.2	47.8	34.3 (29.7–38.8)	54.5 (49.5–59.4)	29.9 (25.3–34.4)
DC	70.3	69.0	19.4	43.8	—	—	—
Florida	66.4	67.2	18.7	44.2	—	—	—
Georgia	67.3	66.6	28.3	52.5	40.3 (39.0–41.6)	56.3 (54.9–57.6)	27.1 (26.0–28.3)
Idaho	66.7	65.0	22.5	44.4	53.6 (50.1–57.1)	65.4 (62.5–68.2)	27.3 (24.4–30.2)
Illinois	71.4	69.3	18.8	49.0	26.9 (24.4–29.4)	55.4 (52.5–58.2)	30.2 (27.9–32.6)
Indiana	65.8	67.1	27.3	50.9	—	—	—
Iowa	74.1	75.4	23.3	48.4	40.5 (37.5–43.3)	49.7 (46.7–52.5)	18.9 (16.5–21.1)
Kansas	72.4	75.0	27.8	46.4	33.2 (30.2–36.0)	58.7 (55.5–61.5)	27.7 (24.9–30.4)
Kentucky	69.8	73.3	38.1	58.9	28.8 (26.0–31.6)	59.8 (57.1–62.6)	34.6 (31.9–37.4)
Louisiana	66.3	66.6	31.4	52.7	—	—	—
Maine	68.7	69.3	24.3	49.9	47.7 (44.9–50.4)	44.8 (42.0–47.4)	20.5 (18.3–22.6)
Maryland	74.8	73.6	16.7	43.5	23.7 (19.0–28.4)	42.4 (37.5–47.3)	25.9 (21.6–30.2)
Massachusetts	78.2	79.0	16.5	41.6	53.8 (49.5–58.0)	48.2 (45.0–51.4)	25.8 (22.4–29.2)
Michigan	75.9	75.3	17.2	43.0	23.3 (19.7–26.9)	58.0 (54.8–61.2)	25.0 (21.4–28.6)
Minnesota	79.0	78.7	14.3	38.3	—	—	—
Mississippi	58.0	56.6	29.6	58.2	25.6 (24.3–26.8)	68.9 (67.5–70.2)	39.1 (37.7–40.5)
Missouri	63.4	63.0	25.2	49.4	28.6 (27.6–29.6)	54.7 (53.6–55.8)	27.0 (26.0–28.0)
Montana	64.7	60.6	19.6	42.6	—	—	—

	Dental visit	Teeth cleaning	Edentulism	Six or more teeth lost	Sealants	Caries	Untreated caries
Nebraska	74.3	75.0	43.7	23.1	45.3 (41.3–49.2)	59.3 (55.0–63.6)	17.0 (13.6–20.4)
Nevada	62.0	63.2	47.1	16.5	33.2 (27.5–38.9)	67.1 (64.2–70.1)	39.0 (35.0–43.1)
New Hampshire	76.2	77.9	45.8	21.1	46.0 (37.7–54.0)	52.1 (45.5–58.4)	21.8 (14.3–29.1)
New Jersey	74.4	74.8	44.1	17.0	—	—	—
New Mexico	66.4	66.3	43.0	21.8	43.3 (34.6–51.8)	64.7 (59.5–69.7)	37.1 (32.3–41.6)
New York	70.0	70.4	46.8	16.9	27.0 (21.3–32.7)	54.1 (51.5–56.6)	33.1 (29.6–36.6)
North Carolina	67.7	69.5	55.0	28.3	52.8 (49.6–55.8)	55.7 (52.5–58.7)	17.0 (14.7–19.4)
North Dakota	68.4	67.6	49.3	25.0	—	—	—
Ohio	71.3	71.1	47.3	20.4	—	—	—
Oklahoma	60.5	59.4	55.5	31.2	37.3 (32.8–41.5)	69.5 (65.1–73.4)	40.3 (35.8–44.7)
Oregon	67.1	66.0	43.0	17.8	50.8 (46.5–55.0)	60.7 (57.4–64.0)	22.1 (18.7–25.5)
Pennsylvania	68.4	69.6	52.7	23.8	26.1 (23.1–29.1)	52.6 (49.2–55.9)	27.3 (23.9–30.6)
Puerto Rico	67.3	70.6	62.9	24.5	—	—	—
Rhode Island	77.3	78.8	43.2	18.4	—	—	—
South Carolina	66.7	66.7	49.7	21.8	20.3 (19.6–21.1)	57.9 (57.0–58.9)	32.5 (31.6–33.4)
South Dakota	71.3	70.2	54.2	26.1	49.6 (44.2–55.0)	66.9 (60.8–73.0)	30.2 (22.8–37.5)
Tennessee	69.0	71.5	53.6	32.3	—	—	—
Texas	59.2	58.7	39.4	16.8	—	—	—
Utah	71.6	69.3	32.6	13.6	50.1 (46.0–54.0)	61.1 (59.0–64.0)	23.1 (21.0–25.0)
Vermont	73.2	74.5	47.8	21.3	66.1 (59.4–72.9)	45.1 (39.0–51.1)	16.2 (12.9–19.5)
Virgin Islands	59.0	55.4	45.1	14.7	—	—	—
Virginia	72.8	71.8	43.4	19.4	—	—	—
Washington	70.0	69.3	39.1	16.1	50.4 (46.8–54.1)	59.7 (56.6–62.8)	19.1 (16.7–21.5)
West Virginia	61.5	64.1	69.6	42.9	—	—	—
Wisconsin	76.7	75.7	46.0	19.7	47.1 (45.3–48.7)	60.2 (58.4–61.8)	30.9 (29.3–32.5)
Wyoming	67.0	64.7	46.9	21.8	—	—	—

"—" Indicates data not available; Dental visit: adults aged 18+ who have visited a dentist or dental clinic in the past year (ages 18+); Teeth cleaning: adults aged 18+ who have had their teeth cleaned in the past year (among adults with natural teeth who have ever visited a dentist (ages 18+) or dental clinic); Edentulism: adults aged 65+ who have lost all of their natural teeth because of tooth decay or gum disease (ages 65+); Six or more teeth lost: adults aged 65+ who have lost six or more teeth because of tooth decay or gum disease (ages 65+); Sealants: percentage of 3rd grade students with dental sealants on at least one permanent molar tooth; Caries: percentage of 3rd grade students with caries experience (treated or untreated tooth decay); Untreated caries: percentage of 3rd grade students with untreated tooth decay.

among different dental schools in the United States. In this study, most disagreement was found for deep pockets and for multirooted teeth and disease status; tooth type, age, and full-mouth plaque levels had a significant impact on decision making [12].

Provision of services is a function of availability of the workforce to treat the resident population. However, several pockets may exist where there is a shortage of dentists. The Shortage Designation Branch in the Health Resources and Services Administration (HRSA) Bureau of Health Professions National Center for Health Workforce Analysis develops shortage designation criteria and uses them to decide whether or not a geographic area or population group is a Health Professional Shortage Area or a Medically Underserved Area or Population. HRSA designated Dental Health Professional Shortage areas (D-HPSA), is based on a series of criteria related to geographic area, population count and distribution, dental practitioner count, and is weighted by age and number of dental auxiliaries. A study in Mississippi showed that 55 counties were designated as D-HPSA in 1970, 51 counties in 1980, 30 in 1990, and 40 in 2000 [42]. The study emphasized that although the numbers of D-HPSAs may change with time, substantial oral health disparities remained, and there was a need to monitor practice and D-HPSA designated areas at the state-level to eliminate disparities in oral health.

It is well known that few practices enroll Medicaid patients, which leaves a pool of underserved population within the geographic zone, which might burden other health care delivery settings that may be more expensive to the system and not suitable for the required treatments. For example, a Minnesota report has documented a shift of dental Medicaid patients to using emergency room services, because the Medicaid payment mechanism is not attractive enough for practices to incorporate the public program into its fold [43].

Gilbert and colleagues [10] reported that tooth-specific case-mix adjustment in practices explains social disparity variation in tooth loss. They further reported that Blacks and those persons with a lower socio-economic position were more likely to receive a dental extraction once they enter the dental care system, given the same disease extent and severity in the Florida dental study.

Predictors of oral health disparities

Oral health is predicted not only by childhood socioeconomic position, but also by oral health in childhood; that is, different events during the life-course of an individual interplay in different ways to result in observed disparities [44]. Conducting a longstanding cohort study of 789 subjects who had tooth loss at ages 5 and 26 years, Thomson and colleagues [44] found that after controlling for childhood oral health, those with a lower socio-economic position at 5 years of age had substantially greater caries experience (mean decayed and filled surface and mean decayed surface scores). The investigators found that by the time subjects reached 26 years of age, more were likely to have lost a tooth in adulthood because of caries and also had a greater prevalence and extent of periodontitis. It is likely that barriers to better oral health, if they persist, continue to act in similar predictable ways. This could lead to a cumulative effect on not only increasing the burden of disease, but also on the ability to access and use the oral health care system, thereby altering the responsiveness to oral health problems.

Responsiveness to new dental symptoms may play a significant role in initiating and maintaining oral health disparities. The Florida dental study noted that, whereas Blacks and persons of lower socio-economic position reported more new dental symptoms, they were less likely to obtain dental care to address these symptoms. When they did receive care, they were more likely to experience tooth loss and less likely to report that dentists had discussed alternative treatments with them [10]. Although some of this attitude may be attributed to cultural and behavioral characteristics of the population, persistent lower socio-economic position may work through a lack of information, inability to pay for alternative treatment modalities, and low self-confidence, resulting in under-use of the oral health care delivery system. A prospective cohort study, using in-person and telephonic interviews, found that even after adjusting for key predisposing, enabling, and oral health need characteristics, Blacks were less likely to seek dental care during follow-up, more likely to be problem-oriented dental attendees, be unable to pay an unexpected $500 dental bill, and to report subsequent dental problems [45]. Examining these factors further, this study noted that frustration with past dental care, propensity to use a homemade remedy, and lack of dental insurance were significant predictors among Blacks. However, these factors were not significant predictors among non-Hispanic Whites, who were more likely to seek care for preventive reasons [45,46].

In an attempt to explain the failure of the oral health care delivery system to increase use or insurance coverage, despite a period of exemplary and sustained economic boom, it has been suggested that a possible self-selection process may be occurring, where only those members of the population who believe they have sufficient resources actually seek care in the fee-charging system [30]. Strategies will need to be developed and implemented in ways that circumvent the apparent unresponsiveness of the dental care system to economic effects of market forces [30] if the disparities are to be eliminated, to reach a goal of yet to be defined equitable optimal oral health.

Steps to eliminate oral health disparities

With substantial existing oral health disparities, the ethics of dental practice and the profession are being called into question to answer the question, "Who will provide the necessary leadership to address and resolve these issues, so that oral health is attainable by all?" [47]. As with general health disparities [1], oral health disparities also work through a complex web of multilevel interacting factors [48]. Interaction of these factors across different levels will need to be understood carefully to develop workable plans to eliminate disparities, especially under the dynamic population change toward a more mixed and multiethnic society that the United States and most other countries are expected to witness. Some suggestions to address oral health disparities at different levels include: increasing workforce diversity [49]; a military-style oral health care system (members of the United States military have universal access to care that also has a compulsory component) [50]; developing networks comprising community- and faith-based organizations, local and national government health institutions, clinical service providers, researchers, and immigrant-service and advocacy organizations [51]; increasing minority-oriented research activities [52]; modifying clinical timings to accommodate work-hours and other time commitments of those with poorer oral health status [53]; and direct involvement of community representatives in community-based participatory research [54].

It has often been proposed that increasing the number of underrepresented minorities in the work force to serve the needs of growing minority populations will contribute substantially toward eliminating oral health disparities. Such proposals are based on an assumption that minority patients prefer or would prefer to be treated by providers of the same race and ethnicity as themselves (the racial concordance hypothesis). Based on a randomized trial to test this racial concordance hypothesis in a dental school setting, Bender [55] reported that overall, 58% of the participants had no preference for the race or gender of their student dentist. This study also reported that Hispanic women were especially likely to prefer racial and gender concordance. Although the investigators concluded that "the racial concordance hypothesis may not apply to choosing a dentist and thus may not be as strong an argument to justify efforts to increase diversity in dental schools as previously thought" [55], the study did not assess adjustment for several other factors that could have affected the outcomes, such as the role of various socio-economic factors, language barriers, educational level of patients, and other factors.

Whereas the search for all modifiable factors influencing oral health disparities is on, several states have started to take steps to assess and address oral health disparities in their jurisdictions, as outlined below.

Initiate studies to identify and document existing disparities in the population

Develop goals, a plan, and a road map to address oral health disparities

Identify current infrastructural capacity and plan for future expanded goals

Initiate oral health surveillance systems to monitor the oral health condition of the population and monitor disparities

Expand and maintain the state's oral disease preventive services through programs such as water fluoridation, dental sealants, health education, and school-based programs through fixed and mobile clinics

Develop oral health prevention programs for adults and children in remote areas, through various centering initiatives

Develop tobacco habit prevention programs

Find alternatives for improving access to oral health care through increasing program, service, and insurance coverage

Maintain a regular oral health surveillance system, using existing self-report surveys and news surveys where necessary

Eliminating disparities in oral health will require enhanced efforts at preventing disease, promoting health, and delivering appropriate care. It will also require a thorough understanding of the lower use of already available effective preventive and treatment services, and additional interventions to address the identified causes [56]. Assessing a State's poor performance on oral health indicators, a recent report suggested allocation of additional resources to increase oral health awareness, create and maintain preventive programs, improve the social insurance programs, increase the availability of providers in rural areas, and encourage practitioners to serve the poor by improving the reimbursement of social entitlement programs [57]. Such support-led policies may be able to help under-performing states to overcome disparities and at least achieve targeted levels of oral health indicators, as outlined in the Healthy People 2010 objectives.

Oral health disparities are an international phenomenon, and perhaps a global action of learning from the experiences of other countries will provide deeper insights into its mechanisms and possible solutions. This thought was best summarized by Maas [58]: "... while public funding and the public provision of services (such as programs in schools or community health centers) can be powerful instruments of change, they have their limitations. Examination of all types of public subsidization of dental care may reveal inadvertent distributions that may increase disparities. The discovery of best practices and lessons learned in the financing and organization of dental care may begin by comparing US experiences with those of other countries."

Summary

Oral health disparities in the United States refers to the existence of differences in the incidence, prevalence, mortality, and burden of oral diseases and other adverse health conditions, as well as use of health care services among specific population groups in the country. The first ever Surgeon General's report on oral health, Oral Health in America—A report of the Surgeon General in 2000, set out the agenda identifying the need for research, identifying, and eliminating or reducing oral health disparities in the United States. Existence of disparities in oral health status, accessing and using the oral health care delivery system, and receiving treatment depending on gender, race or ethnicity, education, income, disability, geographic location, and sexual orientation have been documented. NIDCR has laid out a list of groups to be targeted for the elimination or reduction of oral health disparities, and different states have initiated a series of steps as tools to document, assess, develop strategies, and monitor progress in efforts to eliminate or reduce oral health disparities in the United States.

References

[1] Sen A, Dreze J. The Amartya Sen and Jean Dreze Omnibus. New Delhi: Oxford University Press; 1999.
[2] The Sveriges Riksbank prize in economic sciences in memory of Alfred Nobel 1998. Presentation speech by Professor Robert Erikson of the Royal Academy of Sciences. Available at: http://nobelprize.org/nobel_prizes/economics/laureates/1998/presentation-speech.html. Accessed January 2, 2008.
[3] NIH. Strategic research plan and budget to reduce and ultimately eliminate health disparities. vol 1. Fiscal Years 2002–2006.
[4] National Cancer Institute. Defining health disparities. Available at: http://seer.cancer.gov/publications/disparities/md_defining.pdf. Accessed January 2, 2008.
[5] Minority Health and Health Disparities Research and Education Act of 2000, Public Law 106–525.
[6] U.S. Department of Health and Human Services. Oral health in America: a report of the Surgeon General. Rockville (MD): U.S. Department of Health and Human Services, National Institute of Dental and Craniofacial Research, National Institutes of Health; 2000.
[7] 07.NIDCR. Health Disparities program. A plan to eliminate craniofacial, oral and dental health disparities. Available at: http://www.nidcr.nih.gov/Research/Extramural/ClinicalResearch/HealthDisparitiesProgram.htm. Accessed January 2, 2008.
[8] Kressin NR. Racial/Ethnic disparities in health care: lessons from medicine for dentistry. J Dent Educ 2005;69(9):998–1002.
[9] O'Neill E. Dental practice patterns add to oral health disparity. J Calif Dent Assoc 2002; 30(12):883–4.
[10] Gilbert GH, Duncan RP, Shelton BJ. Social determinants of tooth loss. Health Serv Res 2003;38(6 Pt 2):1843–62.
[11] Gilbert GH. Racial and socioeconomic disparities in health from population-based research to practice-based research: the example of oral health. J Dent Educ 2005;69(9):1003–14.
[12] Cosyn J, De Bruyn H. Interclinician disparity in periodontal decision making: need for consensus statements on surgical treatment. J Periodontal Res 2007;42(4):311–7.
[13] Dye BA, Tan S, Smith V, et al. Trends in oral health status: United States, 1988–1994 and 1999–2004. Vital Health Stat 11 2007;(248):1–92.
[14] Beltrán-Aguilar ED, Barker LK, Canto MT, et al. Surveillance for dental caries, dental sealants, tooth retention, edentulism, and enamel fluorosis—United States, 1988–1994 and 1999–2002. MMWR Surveill Summ 2005;54(3):1–43.
[15] Vargas CM, Ronzio CR. Disparities in early childhood caries. BMC Oral Health 2006; 6(Suppl 1):S3.
[16] Edelstein BL. Disparities in oral health and access to care: findings of national surveys. Ambul Pediatr 2002;2(2 Suppl):141–7.
[17] Cunha-Cruz J, Hujoel PP, Nadanovsky P. Secular trends in socio-economic disparities in edentulism: USA, 1972–2001. J Dent Res 2007;86(2):131–6.

[18] Gilbert GH, Shewchuk RM, Litaker MS. Effect of dental practice characteristics on racial disparities in patient-specific tooth loss. Med Care 2006;44(5):414–20.

[19] Craig RG, Yip JK, Mijares DQ, et al. Progression of destructive periodontal diseases in three urban minority populations: role of clinical and demographic factors. J Clin Periodontol 2003;30(12):1075–83.

[20] Borrell LN, Taylor GW, Borgnakke WS, et al. Factors influencing the effect of race on established periodontitis prevalence. J Public Health Dent 2003;63(1):20–9.

[21] Dye BA, Vargas CM. The use of a modified CPITN approach to estimate periodontal treatment needs among adults aged 20–79 years by socio-demographic characteristics in the United States, 1988–94. Community Dent Health 2002;19(4):215–23.

[22] Morse DE, Kerr AR. Disparities in oral and pharyngeal cancer incidence, mortality and survival among Black and White Americans. J Am Dent Assoc 2006;137(2):203–12.

[23] Tomar SL, Loree M, Logan H. Racial differences in oral and pharyngeal cancer treatment and survival in Florida. Cancer Causes Control 2004;15(6):601–9.

[24] Miller CS, Henry RG, Rayens MK. Disparities in risk of and survival from oropharyngeal squamous cell carcinoma. Oral Surg Oral Med Oral Pathol Oral Radiol Endod 2003;95(5): 570–5.

[25] Elter JR, Patton LL, Strauss RP. Incidence rates and trends for oral and pharyngeal cancer in North Carolina: 1990–1999. Oral Oncol 2005;41(5):470–9 [Epub 2005 Mar 16].

[26] Riley JL 3rd, Gilbert GH, Heft MW. Socioeconomic and demographic disparities in symptoms of orofacial pain. J Public Health Dent 2003;63(3):166–73.

[27] Riley JL 3rd, Gilbert GH, Heft MW. Orofacial pain: racial and sex differences among older adults. J Public Health Dent 2002;62(3):132–9.

[28] Pezzementi ML, Fisher MA. Oral health status of people with intellectual disabilities in the southeastern United States. J Am Dent Assoc 2005;136(7):903–12.

[29] Havercamp SM, Scandlin D, Roth M. Health disparities among adults with developmental disabilities, adults with other disabilities, and adults not reporting disability in North Carolina. Public Health Rep 2004;119(4):418–26.

[30] Chattopadhyay A, Kumar JV, Green EL. The New York State Minority Health Survey: determinants of oral health care utilization. J Public Health Dent 2003;63(3): 158–65.

[31] Hughes DC, Duderstadt KG, Soobader MP, et al. Disparities in children's use of oral health services. Public Health Rep 2005;120(4):455–62.

[32] CDC. National oral health surveillance system. Available at: http://www.cdc.gov/nohss/. Accessed January 2, 2008.

[33] Centers for Disease Control and Prevention. Dental service use and dental insurance coverage — United States, behavioral risk factor surveillance system. MMWR Morb Mortal Wkly Rep 1997;46(No.50):1199–203.

[34] Nelson S, Armogan V, Abel Y, et al. Disparity in orthodontic utilization and treatment need among high school students. J Public Health Dent 2004;64(1):26–30.

[35] Kressin NR, Boehmer U, Berlowitz D, et al. Racial variations in dental procedures: the case of root canal therapy versus tooth extraction. Med Care 2003;41(11):1256–61.

[36] Borrell LN, Northridge ME, Miller DB, et al. Oral health and health care for older adults: a spatial approach for addressing disparities and planning services. Spec Care Dentist 2006; 26(6):252–6.

[37] Vargas CM, Dye BA, Hayes KL. Oral health status of rural adults in the United States. J Am Dent Assoc 2002;133(12):1672–81.

[38] Zabos GP, Northridge ME, Ro MJ, et al. Lack of oral health care for adults in Harlem: a hidden crisis. Am J Public Health 2002;92(1):49–52.

[39] Chattopadhyay A, Slade GD, Caplan, DJ. Professional charges not reimbursed to dentists in the US: evidence from medical expenditure panel survey, 1996. Community Dent Health (under review).

[40] Tellez M, Sohn W, Burt BA, et al. Assessment of the relationship between neighborhood characteristics and dental caries severity among low-income African-Americans: a multilevel approach. J Public Health Dent 2006;66(1):30–6.

[41] Nash DA, Nagel RJ. Confronting oral health disparities among American Indian/Alaska Native children: the pediatric oral health therapist. Am J Public Health 2005;95(8):1325–9 [Epub 2005 Jul 7].

[42] Krause D, Frate DA, May WL. Demographics and distribution of dentists in Mississippi: a dental work force study. J Am Dent Assoc 2005;136(5):668–77.

[43] Helgeson MJ. The Minnesota oral health care solutions project: implications for people with special needs. J Calif Dent Assoc 2005;33(8):641–9.

[44] Thomson WM, Poulton R, Milne BJ, et al. Socioeconomic inequalities in oral health in childhood and adulthood in a birth cohort. Community Dent Oral Epidemiol 2004;32(5): 345–53.

[45] Gilbert GH, Shah GR, Shelton BJ, et al. Racial differences in predictors of dental care use. Health Serv Res 2002;37(6):1487–507.

[46] Riley JL 3rd, Gilbert GH, Heft MW. Dental attitudes: proximal basis for oral health disparities in adults. Community Dent Oral Epidemiol 2006;34(4):289–98.

[47] Evans CA. Eliminating oral health disparities: ethics workshop reactor comments. J Dent Educ 2006;70(11):1180–3.

[48] Patrick DL, Lee RS, Nucci M, et al. Reducing oral health disparities: a focus on social and cultural determinants. BMC Oral Health 2006;6(Suppl 1):S4.

[49] Mitchell DA, Lassiter SL. Addressing health care disparities and increasing workforce diversity: the next step for the dental, medical, and public health professions. Am J Public Health 2006;96(12):2093–7 [Epub 2006 Oct 31].

[50] Hyman JJ, Reid BC, Mongeau SW, et al. The military oral health care system as a model for eliminating disparities in oral health. J Am Dent Assoc 2006;137(3):372–8.

[51] Gany FM, Shah SM, Changrani J. New York City's immigrant minorities. Reducing cancer health disparities. Cancer 2006;107(8 Suppl):2071–81.

[52] Ramos-Gomez F, Cruz GD, Watson MR, et al. Latino oral health: a research agenda toward eliminating oral health disparities. J Am Dent Assoc 2005;136(9):1231–40.

[53] Kim YO. Reducing disparities in dental care for low-income Hispanic children. J Health Care Poor Underserved 2005;16(3):431–43.

[54] Harrigan RC, Easa D, LeSaux C, et al. Oral health disparities and periodontal disease in Asian and Pacific Island populations. Ethn Dis 2005;15(4 Suppl 5):S5–39–46.

[55] Bender DJ. Patient preference for a racially or gender-concordant student dentist. J Dent Educ 2007;71(6):726–45.

[56] Kumar JV, Green EL. Oral health disparities in New York State. NY State Dent J 2005; 71(7):43–7.

[57] Chattopadhyay A, Arevalo O, Cecil JC 3rd. Kentucky's oral health indicators and progress towards Healthy People 2010 objectives. Ky Med J, in press.

[58] Maas WR. Access to care—what can the United States learn from other countries? Community Dent Oral Epidemiol 2006;34(3):232–40.

THE DENTAL
CLINICS
OF NORTH AMERICA

Dent Clin N Am 52 (2008) 319–332

Multicultural Issues in Oral Health

Raul I. Garcia, DMD, MMedSc*,
Cynthia A. Cadoret, RDH, MPH,
Michelle Henshaw, DDS, MPH

*Department of Health Policy and Health Services Research, Northeast Center
for Research to Evaluate and Eliminate Dental Disparities, Boston University Goldman
School of Dental Medicine, 715 Albany Street, 560, 3rd Floor, Boston, MA 02118, USA*

Demographic changes in American society will have increasingly important effects on the oral health of the nation and on the practice of dentistry. As the French philosopher Auguste Comte (1798–1857) stated, "Demography is destiny." One much discussed demographic trend affecting dentistry is the "graying" of America. According to the United States Census Bureau estimates, by the year 2030 over 20% of Americans will be 65 and older [1]. One consequence of this trend is that in 25 years most of America will appear demographically much like Florida does today. Overall, the number of Americans 65 years or older will double over the coming 35 years, reaching 80 million by the year 2045. The impact on dental practice resulting from these growing numbers of elders has become well recognized.

However, an equally if not more significant demographic trend, but one much less discussed in the context of dental practice, is the dramatic growth in the numbers of Americans from racial and ethnic minority groups. Presently, United States Census statistics show that over 30% of Americans are minorities (ie, Hispanic, African American, Asian, Native American), with Hispanics being the largest of these groups [1]. By 2010, the numbers of minorities are expected to increase to 35%, and by 2025 to approach 40% of the United States population. Another, and related, major demographic trend that also has yet to receive adequate attention in the context of dental practice is the growth in immigration to America.

This work was supported in part by National Institute of Health grants U54 DE-014264 and K24 DE-000419 to Dr. Garcia.

* Corresponding author.
E-mail address: rig@bu.edu (R.I. Garcia).

0011-8532/08/$ - see front matter
doi:10.1016/j.cden.2007.12.006
dental.theclinics.com

From 1990 to 2000 the number of immigrants in the United States increased by 50%, from 20 million to over 30 million. Currently, over 11% of the United States population is foreign-born (over 52% of them are from Latin America and over 26% from Asia). Immigrants represent an even greater proportion of the population in the nation's two largest states: over 20% of California and over 16% of New York. However, the effects of immigration are evident throughout the country; for example, the number of foreign-born in North Carolina, Georgia, and Nevada grew by 200% or more in the past decade. Furthermore, the growth of the foreign-born population segment is expected to accelerate.

The social, political, and economic pressures on the dental profession to meet the health needs of an increasingly diverse society will only grow over the coming decades. It is important to note that within the practicing lifetimes of many current dentists—and certainly of current dental students—the number of persons in our nation who are members of minority groups will exceed the numbers of non-Hispanic Whites in the United States. Our successes as a profession in meeting such challenges are in large part dependent on adequately addressing the multicultural issues that affect doctor-patient communications and patients' health beliefs and attitudes. This is a major field of research activity that is briefly reviewed in this article, with the goal of identifying ways that may enable current and future dental practitioners to become better prepared to meet the needs of such diverse patient populations.

Health disparities and the multicultural imperative

Health disparities are well documented in minority populations, such as African Americans, Hispanics, American Indians, Alaska Natives, and other racial and ethnic minority groups. Individuals in these groups bear a disproportionate burden of disease and disability, and these disparities result in "lower life expectancy, decreased quality of life, loss of economic opportunities, and perceptions of injustice" [2]. In their report addressing ethnic and racial disparities in medical care, Betancourt and colleagues [3] noted that the lack of diversity in both the health care workforce and its leadership has resulted in policies, procedures, and delivery systems that are incapable of serving diverse populations. One simple example includes clinic hours that did not accommodate work schedules, long waiting times to make appointments, and complicated bureaucratic processes. *Unequal Treatment. A Report of the Institute of Medicine* documented the existence of disparities in health care, even when there is equal access to care, and provided evidence of cultural differences in health care between minorities and nonminorities. These differences were also related to disparities in access, health status, and health outcomes [4]. The first United States National Health Care Disparities Report, issued by the Agency for Healthcare

Research and Quality, presented a comprehensive national overview of disparities, including disparities in oral health, and in access to health care services and insurance, health outcomes, and the quality of care among United States racial, ethnic, and socioeconomic groups [2].

A major determinant of oral health disparities is limited access to dental care, both preventive and restorative, and a major barrier to dental care access is lack of dental insurance, in particular private dental coverage [5]. While dental insurance may be an essential prerequisite for ensuring access to care, it may be insufficient by itself for eliminating oral health disparities, as there exist other important determinants of oral health status and dental care access. These may include issues related to doctor-patient communications, including cultural and linguistic competency of care providers and the health beliefs and health literacy of patients [6–8].

Cultural competence in health care may be defined as an understanding of the importance of social and cultural influences on patients' health beliefs and behaviors; considering how these factors interact at multiple levels of the health care delivery system; and, finally, devising interventions that take these issues into account to assure quality health care delivery to diverse patient populations. Inconsistent patient behaviors and attitudes related to compliance with treatment regimens is often a result of cultural conflict between minority patients and their providers. Clinical inexperience in interacting with minority patients and beliefs held by the provider about the behavior or health of minorities may contribute to a cultural dissonance between providers and patients. Additionally, time and resource constraints imposed on clinic visits may result in providers making snap judgments based on prototypes or stereotypic decision-making models when diagnosing and treating patients. Overlooking patients' cultural beliefs may foster a lack of trust in the provider and their diagnoses, and decrease the likelihood that a person will comply with the prescribed treatment.

A related consideration in ensuring appropriate access to culturally competent health care providers is the discordance on the race and ethnicity of patients and providers and the maldistribution of culturally competent providers. A review by the Sullivan Commission's Report on Health Professions Diversity [9] showed that minority patients in the United States have higher levels of satisfaction in race- or ethnicity-concordant settings [10–12]. In a study among the Hispanic population, Flores [13] reported that it was very important to Hispanics to have a physician who speaks Spanish and fully understands Hispanics' cultural values. In a recent study of a Canadian-Asian community, Wang [14] found low accessibility to medical care providers in areas heavily populated by Chinese immigrants. He concluded that such a maldistribution was especially concerning because of the "overwhelmingly strong preference of Chinese immigrants for ethnically and dialectically matched family physicians" [14].

Perceived discrimination affects satisfaction with care and care-seeking behaviors. Such significant effects have also been observed in populations in other countries. In a study of access to medical treatment in Sweden, Wamala and colleagues [15] found that perceived discrimination and socio-economic disadvantage were each independently associated with refraining from use of care. Such perceptions may not only affect patients' care seek-ing, but may also influence dentists' behaviors. In a study from Brazil, Cabral and colleagues [16] found that a patient's race significantly affects dentists' decision-making as to whether to extract or retain a decayed tooth.

Doctor-patient communication may play a major role, as there may be difficulties in communication, particularly in non-English-speaking patients, and in the case of a dentist's or hygienist's inability to speak the patient's native language. But, even among persons of one language group, Spanish, there exist significant variations and Hispanics serve as an example of the complex challenges we face, combining issues of both culture and language, in meeting the needs of both "new Americans" as well as of those who are multigenerational Americans.

Cultural competence is intimately related to health literacy [6–8]. The American Dental Association (ADA) [17] defines oral health literacy as "the degree to which individuals have the capacity to obtain, process, and understand basic health information and services needed to make appropri-ate oral health decisions." Importantly, effective communication is depen-dent on both the oral health literacy of patients as well as the skills, preferences, and expectations of oral health care providers. Health literacy is thoroughly discussed in the article by Dr. Horowitz elsewhere in this issue.

Health behaviors, culture, and oral health

The World Health Organization Constitution [18] presented a holistic definition of health as "a state of complete physical, mental, and social well-being, and not merely the absence of disease or infirmity." From this perspective, the roles and responsibilities of health care professionals go be-yond the biologic and technologic sciences, and enter the sociocultural and behavioral domains of health promotion. Patients' individual preferences and behavioral risk factors are intimately related to their sociodemogra-phic and cultural backgrounds. The resulting oral health beliefs held by patients, and their related risk behaviors, are intimately related to patients' health-related risk behaviors, receptivity to change, and ultimately on pa-tients' health outcomes. To systematically understand oral health outcomes and to design effective oral health interventions, a variety of theoretic frame-works and conceptual models drawn from psychology and social science have been applied to dentistry. For example, Barker [19] has applied the health belief model (HBM) to the analysis of compliance with preventive dental behaviors. The HBM states "that for individuals to follow prescribed advice they must believe that they are susceptible to the disease ('susceptibil-ity'), that the disease is serious ('seriousness'), and that the benefits of following prescribed advice outweigh costs ('benefits')" [19]. Using the HBM, she found that the health beliefs of susceptibility and benefits were significantly related to compliance with preventive dental advice.

It has also been found that oral health risk behaviors may not be modifiable by oral health educational interventions, if such interventions are not framed in a culturally informed and sensitive manner. Nakazono and colleagues [20] used data from the International Collaborative Study of Oral Health Outcomes II USA study to examine oral health beliefs in diverse populations, developing oral health belief measures that corresponded to the HBM dimensions. They found that both age and race-ethnicity were significant predictors of the perceived benefits of preventive practices, with White adults "more likely to believe in the benefit of preventive practices" [20]. Kiyak and colleagues [21], in their study of ethnicity and oral health in older adults, observed that non-White elders tended to have less confidence in their ability to control their oral health. In addition, those elders in their study who were immigrants (primarily the Asian and Hispanic elders) also reported less concern about the value of healthy teeth or "even about saving their natural teeth" [21].

In the authors' own work, the health decision model [22] serves as a useful means by which to conceptualize the interplay of multiple factors (Fig. 1) that affect oral health, including health beliefs. The health decision model is a conceptualization of factors leading to individuals' health decisions and includes a number of potential influences on health decisions, such as health beliefs, individual preferences and knowledge, prior experiences, and social interactions (such as with physicians and family). The application

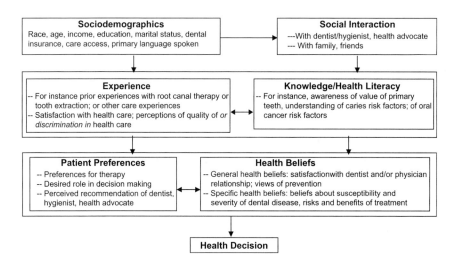

Fig. 1. The health decision model. (*Adapted from* Eraker SA, Kirscht JP, Becker MH. Understanding and improving patient compliance. Ann Intern Med 1984;100:258–68; with permission).

of such a model may serve to guide the design and implementation of health promotion efforts aimed at improving health outcomes in diverse and multicultural populations. For example, it has been found that patients who are more involved in the decisions regarding their treatment have better subsequent health outcomes.

As described by Eraker and colleagues [22], there is not a prespecified causal ordering of factors influencing health decisions. Rather, each of the domains of health beliefs, patient preferences, experience, and knowledge influence one another, and are affected by social interaction and sociodemographic factors as well. Cultural factors, for example such as those related to race, ethnicity, and national origin, will affect each of these domains in variable ways. Thus, the health decision model is not intended to serve as a causal guide for the relationship among these elements, but may instead be used as an organizing framework to design culturally appropriate interventions, as well as to create oral health education and promotion materials that respect cultural beliefs. The materials that are developed may then serve to elevate the oral health literacy of the target population [8] and serve as community resources, patient self-management, and decision support tools.

However, as a "one-size-fits-all" approach will not be maximally effective in multicultural populations, the development of all interventions and materials will most likely need to be adapted and customized to fit the particularities of each cultural group. Thus, while the health decision model has provided a useful framework for much of the authors' work, when it comes to the implementation of a targeted intervention in a culturally diverse setting, the authors have found the chronic care model (CCM) [23] to be a highly relevant conceptual model for implementation and evaluation of interventions in multicultural settings, as described below.

The chronic care model, multicultural factors, and oral health promotion

Given that the most prevalent oral diseases, such as caries and periodontal diseases, are chronic and progressive, yet preventable through behavior modifications, the authors have adopted the CCM (Fig. 2) as the conceptual model guiding the authors' own efforts at addressing oral health disparities. The CCM is driven by a set of organizing principles for basic changes or improvements to support care that is evidence-based, population-based, and patient-centered [23,24]. At its core is the concept of "productive interactions" between the patient and the care provider. The CCM provides a framework in which strategies for improvement can be tailored to local conditions and multicultural actors by considering six fundamental elements (see Fig. 2), including community resources and policies, the health system organization of care, self-management support, an effective delivery system design, decision support, and clinical information systems. The combination

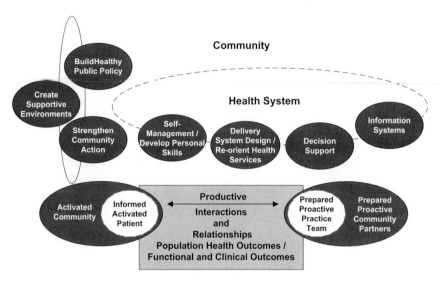

Fig. 2. The expanded chronic care model. (*Adapted from* Barr VJ, Robinson S, Marin-Lonk B, et al. The expanded Chronic Care Model: an integration of concepts and strategies from population health promotion and the Chronic Care Model. Healthcare Q 2003;7:73–82; with permission.)

of these six elements fosters interaction between informed patients and prepared providers that may improve patient outcomes.

Although the CCM was originally developed for improvements in chronic disease management, this and similar models have been posited for applications in prevention [24,25]. Prevention and chronic care activities have several overlapping characteristics, such as behavioral counseling and preventive checks that allow for this dual application. Furthermore, activities such as patient-centered care underscore both chronic disease management and prevention efforts that facilitate positive health behaviors and improved outcomes [26].

Implementing solutions in a multicultural context

Underserved populations encounter numerous barriers when attempting to access both preventive dental care and restorative dental services. These barriers to health care may be significantly reduced by community-based interventions through the work of a peer health advocate, or a lay-person health promoter (promotora) [27], who best understands the cultural perspectives of the population. Community health workers (CHW) are defined as "community members who work almost exclusively in community settings and serve as connectors between health care consumers and providers to promote health among groups that have traditionally lacked access to adequate care" [28]. Expanding the role of such CHWs to include oral health promotion will be valuable in meeting the needs of diverse groups. CHW programs are proven, cost-effective interventions that are used to expand health access and health care services to underserved and underinsured minority communities [29]. They have been used extensively to reach diverse populations, such as migrant farm workers, mothers and infants, African Americans, and Hispanic or Latino populations.

The "promotora" is a CHW model, customized for Latino populations, that has been shown to be effective in reducing chronic disease risk factors through education, dietary interventions, and increasing screening rates. The extent of success seems to be dependent on the autonomy of individual promotoras and the support of partnering community based organizations. For example, a community based outreach program, "Salud para su Corazon" (Health for Your Heart) tested the efficacy of the promotora model for promoting heart health and reducing cardio vascular disease risk factors within seven Latino communities across the country [29]. This model was shown to be highly successful in increasing heart healthy knowledge and behaviors.

One study of the impact of a promotora on increasing compliance with annual preventive exams in uninsured women, aged 40 and over and living at the Mexico-United States border, showed that using a promotora increased compliance with routine screening exams and was highly effective for reaching this Hispanic population [30]. However, in their evaluation of the effect of promotoras and tailored health information materials on dietary intervention in Hispanics, Elder and colleagues [31] found that the effect was not sustained over time once the intervention by the promotora stopped, suggesting that continuity of effort in such communities is needed for sustained improvements.

A related issue is the importance of diversity in the health care professions, whose enhancement is increasingly recognized as being vital to successfully addressing the health needs of a diverse population [9]. A review of the evidence for the value of diversity in the health care workforce concluded that greater racial and ethnic diversity among health professionals will improve access to and quality of health care for all Americans [9,32]. Formicola and colleagues [33] examined these issues as they relate to oral health and suggest that in dentistry as in medicine, when financial access barriers are eliminated then similar cultural factors may account for disparities in oral health. They identified various factors (at the systems level, patient level, and provider level), separate from health care access, that affect disparities in treatments and outcomes between minorities and nonminorities [33].

Patient-centered care and cultural competence

In addition to the need to use culturally and linguistically competent community residents to promote oral health, it is also clear that dental professionals themselves must gain proficiency in providing culturally competent care [3,33] and in enhancing the oral health literacy [8] of the communities they serve. Patient-centered care, as defined by the Institute of Medicine [34], is providing "care that is respectful of and responsive to individual patient preferences, needs, and values and ensuring that patient values guide all clinical decisions." It is thus self-evident that for such care to be maximally effective it must also be provided in a culturally competent manner. To ensure the highest quality care, patients need to be actively involved in decisions about their care and to receive treatment focused on their needs and preferences, as well as advice and counsel from providers of care [26,34]. It has become well recognized that patient-provider communication, and the interactions between provider and patient, play a crucial role in the effectiveness of treatment and in achieving desired outcomes [3,26,34].

In a study assessing patient-centered care on primary care outcomes, Stewart and colleagues [26] found that patient-centered communication was correlated with patients feeling that they were actively engaged in their treatment and finding "common ground" with their physician. Additionally, positive perceptions were associated with better recovery from their chief concern, better emotional health subsequent to the visit, and fewer diagnostic tests and referrals. Effective patient-provider communication results in greater patient satisfaction with the care that they receive, an increase in patient compliance with treatment, and consequently better outcomes. The elements of effective patient-provider communication include [35]:

- Build a relationship
- Open the discussion
- Gather information
- Understand the patient's perspective
- Share information
- Reach agreement on problems and plans
- Provide closure

Difficulties in communication based on the patient and provider speaking different languages may be addressed by using trained interpreters who facilitate communication between patients and health care providers and staff. Culturally competent care and use of professional interpreter services were positively correlated with perceptions of quality of care in a study of Asian-American patients with limited English language skills [36]. Most importantly, effective communication is essential to achieve positive health behaviors, reduce risk factors, and improve outcomes.

However, while overcoming cultural and language barriers is a necessary prerequisite, it is not always sufficient. In cases where even the best culturally competent care is practiced, challenges may arise when there is a need to enhance motivation to change health behaviors in patients who are not motivated to change. In those situations, there may be great value in applying a specific motivational intervention, such as "motivational interviewing" [37], to enhance patients' motivation to change health behaviors in those patients who are resistant or not motivated to change. This intervention is patient-centered and is directly tailored to patients' readiness to change behavior. For those patients at lower motivational levels, techniques such as cognitive dissonance (highlighting the discrepancy between actual and ideal states), exploring outcome expectations, decisional balance (reviewing the costs and benefits of change), and helping the patient understand the detrimental role that the unhealthy behavior plays in his or her life, are important. Helping the patient work through their ambivalence about health behavior change is also essential. Increasingly, more directive approaches are used for those at higher motivational levels, such as skill building, increasing self-efficacy for making change, helping with decision-making, and preventing relapse. Motivational interviewing has been applied to a variety of health behaviors, including alcohol use, smoking, diet, physical activity, pain management, health screening, sexual behavior, medication adherence, as well as to oral health promotion.

Cultural competence, service learning, and dental education

The education of culturally competent practitioners should ideally be started early in dental students' training and be an integral part of the curriculum over all years of dental school. Hewlett and colleagues [38] assessed dental students' perceptions of the adequacy of the cultural competency training they received in dental school, and found that 25% of graduating seniors felt time devoted to cultural competency was inadequate. Almost half of the students also reported that there was inadequate time devoted to other clinical disciplines (implant dentistry, orthodontics) and practice management. With this in mind, it was concluded that integrating cultural competence into the existing curriculum would be more effective than adding separate courses on cultural competence [39]. In addition, key components of such curricular integration should include education on the nature of health disparities and on the social responsibility of health professionals to provide care to the underserved.

Service learning is a method of learning that couples learning with service, with an emphasis on the student's reflection of the experience, and is especially valuable in addressing multicultural issues in dental education and dental care [39,40]. The gains are on many levels. The student is able to apply what has been learned in school to "real life" in treating patients. In addition, the setting may be such that the student is immersed in an underserved community and is able to experience the challenge of treating culturally diverse patient groups who may also have limited resources to afford dental care. The key component to service learning is the reflection requirement, whereby students are encouraged to reflect on the experience by either keeping a journal or doing a structured, supervised project.

In 2003, the Robert Wood Johnson Foundation launched a multimillion dollar program, "Pipeline, Profession and Practice: Community-based Dental Education." With the goal to enhance system capacity, it has aimed to promote community-based dental education, educate culturally competent practitioners, expand access to care in underserved communities, and increase the numbers of underrepresented minority and disadvantaged students in dental schools.

A greater challenge involves the educational needs of current practitioners to provide care in a culturally competent manner and to address health disparities. One way to meet this need may be to design and offer "service learning" continuing education courses for participating in a community-based dental program. However, there appear to be few such opportunities for continuing education in cultural competency aimed at practicing dentists and hygienists, although there is a growing realization of the need and such a course was offered at the 2007 ADA annual session.

Summary

This article has reviewed the importance of multicultural factors in affecting oral health outcomes. In this regard, the cultural competence of oral health care providers merits examination as one point of intervention, to the extent that trust in and comfort with one's dentist is important to effective use of care and adoption of preventive and positive health behaviors. There is a clear need in dentistry for enhancing the cultural competence and communications skills of care providers. In addition, to adequately address the needs of a diverse population and to improve health outcomes, we also need to consider several other challenges. Some specific areas in dentistry that may require attention, or that may need to be newly incorporated into dental care, may include changes in the types of practitioners who comprise the oral health workforce, as well as other improvements in the structure and processes of care. One such approach may be to examine the benefits of "open access" or "advanced access" scheduling as one means by which to promote culturally appropriate care in a logistically feasible manner [41,42].

The effectiveness of CHWs, such as promotoras, was also discussed. There has been increasing interest in the role of primary care medical practitioners in oral health promotion. The potential roles of CHWs and others in community-based oral health care need to be more broadly considered as essential contributors to addressing multicultural factors and oral health disparities. Similarly, creative solutions are needed on the best ways in which to expand the dental team and thereby extend, safely and effectively, the ability of dentists to promote oral health, and to prevent and treat disease in diverse multicultural populations with oral health disparities. Lastly, it is becoming increasingly clear that enhancing the cultural diversity of the health care workforce, including oral health care providers, will be vital to successfully addressing the health needs of our nation's increasingly diverse population [9,32].

Acknowledgments

We thank our colleagues in the Northeast Center for Research to Evaluate and Eliminate Dental Disparities (The CREEDD) for their many contributions. In particular, we acknowledge the input of Brenda Heaton MPH, and Paul Geltman MD, for their insights on conceptual models for health behavior change and health literacy as they relate to oral health promotion and disease prevention in diverse populations.

References

[1] US Census Bureau. The 2008 statistical abstract, National Data Book. Available at: http://www.census.gov/compendia/statab/cats/population.html. Accessed January 29, 2008.

[2] Agency for Healthcare Research and Quality. National Healthcare Disparities Report, 2003, US DHHS Pub. No. 04–0035. Rockville (MD): AHRQ.

[3] Betancourt JR, Green AR, Carrillo JE, et al. Defining cultural competence: a practical framework for addressing racial/ethnic disparities in health and health care. Public Health Rep 2003;118:293–302.

[4] Smedley BD, Stith AY, Nelson AR, editors. Unequal treatment: confronting racial and ethnic disparities in health care. Washington (DC): National Academies Press; 2003. p. 782.

[5] Manski RJ, Macek MD, Moeller JF. Private dental coverage: who has it and how does it influence dental visits and expenditures? J Am Dent Assoc 2002;133:1551–9.

[6] Nielsen-Bohlman L, Panzer AM, Kindig DA, editors. Health literacy: a prescription to end confusion. Washington (DC): National Academies Press; 2004. p. 368.

[7] Agency for Healthcare Research and Quality. Literacy and Health Outcomes. Rockville (MD): AHRQ Evidence Report/Technology Assessment No. 87. AHRQ Publ. No. 04-E007-2, 2004, USDHHS.

[8] National Institute of Dental and Craniofacial Research, National Institute of Health, U.S. Public Health Service, Department of Health and Human Services. The invisible barrier: literacy and its relationship with oral health. J Public Health Dent 2005;65(3):174–82.

[9] Sullivan LW. Missing persons: minorities in the health professions. A Report of the Sullivan Commission on Diversity in the Healthcare Workforce. 2004; WT Kellogg Foundation, p. 201.

[10] LaVeist TA, Nuru-Jeter A. Is doctor-patient race concordance associated with greater satisfaction with care? J Health Soc Behav 2002;43(3):296–306.

[11] LaVeist TA, Carroll T. Race of physician and satisfaction with care among African American patients. J Natl Med Assoc 2002;94(11):937–43.

[12] Saha S, Komaromy M, Koepsell TD, et al. Patient-physician racial concordance and the perceived quality and use of health care. Arch Intern Med 1999;159:997–1004.

[13] Flores G. Culture and the patient-physician relationship: achieving cultural competency in health care. J Pediatr 2004;136(1):14–23.

[14] Wang L. Immigration, ethnicity, and accessibility to culturally diverse family physicians. Health Place 2007;13:656–71.

[15] Wamala S, Merlo J, Bostrom G, et al. Perceived discrimination, socioeconomic disadvantage and refraining from seeking medical treatment in Sweden. J Epidemiol Community Health 2007;61:409–15.

[16] Cabral ED, Caldas AF Jr, Cabral HAM. Influence of the patient's race on the dentist's decision to extract or retain a decayed tooth. Community Dent Oral Epidemiol 2005;33: 461–6.

[17] American Dental Association. ADA community brief: oral health literacy. Available at: http://www.ada.org/prof/resources/pubs/epubs/brief/brief_0711.htm. Accessed December 3, 2007.

[18] Constitution of the World Health Organization. WHO Basic Documents. 45th edition. Supplement. Geneva (Switzerland): World Health Organization; October 2006. Available at: http://www.who.int/governance/eb/who_constitution_en.pdf. Accessed December 3, 2007.

[19] Barker T. Role of health beliefs in patient compliance with preventive dental advice. Community Dent Oral Epidemiol 1994;22:327–30.

[20] Nakazono TT, Davidson PL, Andersen RM. Oral health beliefs in diverse populations. Adv Dent Res 1997;11:235–44.

[21] Kiyak HA, Kamoh A, Persson RE, et al. Ethnicity and oral health in community-dwelling older adults. Gen Dent 2002;50:513–8.

[22] Eraker SA, Kirscht JP, Becker MH. Understanding and improving patient compliance. Ann Intern Med 1984;100:258–68.

[23] Wagner EH, Davis C, Shaefer J, et al. A survey of leading chronic disease management programs: are they consistent with the literature? Manag Care Q 1999;7:56–66.

[24] Barr VJ, Robinson S, Marin-Lonk B, et al. The expanded Chronic Care Model: an integration of concepts and strategies from population health promotion and the Chronic Care Model. Hosp Q 2003;7:73–82.

[25] Gooch BF, Malvitz DM, Griffin SO, et al. Promoting the oral health of older adults through the chronic disease model: CDC's perspective on what we still need to know. J Dent Educ 2005;69:1058–63.

[26] Stewart M, Brown JB, Donner A, et al. The impact of patient-centered care on outcomes. J Fam Pract 2000;49:796–804.

[27] Watson MR, Horowitz A, Garcia I, et al. A community participatory oral health promotion program in an inner-city Latino community. J Public Health Dent 2001;61:34–41.

[28] Witmer A, Seifer SD, Finocchio L, et al. Community health workers: integral members of the health care work force. Am J Public Health 1995;85(8):1055–8.

[29] Balcazar H, Alvarado M, Hollen ML, et al. Evaluation of Salud Para Su Corazon (Health for Your Heart)—National Council of La Raza Promotora outreach program. Prev Chronic Dis [serial online] 2005 July. Available at: http://www.cdc.gov/pcd/issues/2005/jul/04_0130. htm. Accessed December 3, 2007.

[30] Hunter JB, Guernsey de Zapien J, Papenfuss M, et al. The impact of a promotora on increasing routine chronic disease prevention among women aged 40 and older at the U.S.-Mexico border. Health Educ Behav 2004;31:18S–28S.

[31] Elder JP, Ayala GX, Campbell NR, et al. Long-term effects of a communication intervention for Spanish-dominant Latinas. Am J Prev Med 2006;31(2):159–66.

[32] Smedley BD, Stith-Butler A, Bristow LR, editors. In the nation's compelling interest: ensuring diversity in the health-care workforce. Washington (DC): National Academies Press; 2004. p. 432.

[33] Formicola AJ, Stavisky J, Lewy R. Cultural competency: dentistry and medicine learning from one another. J Dent Educ 2003;67:869–75.

[34] Committee on Quality of Health Care in America, Institute of Medicine. Crossing the Quality Chasm: a New Health System for the 21st Century. Washington (DC): National Academy Press; 2001. p. 360.

[35] Makoul G. Essential elements of communication in medical encounters: the Kalamazoo Consensus Statement. Acad Med 2001;76(4):390–3.

[36] Ngo-Metzger Q, Massagli MP, Clarridge BR, et al. Linguistic and cultural barriers to care. Perspectives of Chinese and Vietnamese immigrants. J Gen Intern Med 2003;18:44–52.

[37] Miller WR, Rollnick S. Motivational interviewing: preparing people for change. 2nd edition. New York: The Guilford Press; 2002. p. 428.

[38] Hewlett ER, Davidson PL, Nakazono TT, et al. Effect of school environment on dental students' perceptions of cultural competency curricula and preparedness to care for diverse populations. J Dent Educ 2007;71:810–8.

[39] Yoder KM. A framework for service-learning in dental education. J Dent Educ 2006;70: 115–23.

[40] Henshaw M. Service-learning. Oral health disparities and the shift in dental education. In: Welie JVM, editor. Justice in oral health care. Ethical and educational perspectives. (Marquette studies in philosophy; no 47). Milwaukee (WI): Marquette University Press; 2006. p. 261–83.

[41] O'Connor ME, Matthews BS, Gao D. Effect of open access scheduling on missed appointments, immunizations, and continuity of care for infant well-child care visits. Arch Pediatr Adolesc Med 2006;160:889–93.

[42] Murray M, Bodenheimer T, Rittenhouse D, et al. Improving timely access to primary care. JAMA 2003;289:1042–6.

ELSEVIER
SAUNDERS

THE DENTAL
CLINICS
OF NORTH AMERICA

Dent Clin N Am 52 (2008) 333–344

Oral Health Literacy: The New Imperative to Better Oral Health

Alice M. Horowitz, PhD*,
Dushanka V. Kleinman, DDS, MScD

*School of Public Health, University of Maryland, 3310 HHP Building,
College Park, MD 20742, USA*

*Have you ever experienced a misunderstanding with a patient about a given
procedure or the outcome of a procedure? Has a patient ever called your office
to clarify the self-care instructions after an appointment?*

Effective communication with patients—speaking and presenting information in a clear and appropriate format and active listening—is essential
to quality dental care and can contribute to successful oral health outcomes.
Oral health outcomes are a product of numerous factors that contribute to
oral health promotion and disease prevention. Factors, such as professional
clinical dental care and appropriate self-care, play a key role, as do community initiatives like community water fluoridation and school dental sealant
programs. To benefit from the many preventive measures that exist and to
navigate through the health care system, patients need to be aware of the
measures and the additional required services, know where to access
them, and know how to use them appropriately. While patients obtain information from multiple sources, the clinical care and information provided to
them by their dentist and dental team members serve to guide and inform
their ability for optimum oral health self-care and decision-making related
to health overall. The encounter with a dentist or dental hygienist is an opportunity for patients to receive guidance and learn skills for their self-care
and for additional health services they may require. The communication
skills of the dental team contribute to a patient's health literacy that contributes to improved health outcomes.

* Corresponding author. 4501 Walsh Street, Chevy Chase, MD 20815.
E-mail address: ahorowit@umd.edu (A.M. Horowitz).

0011-8532/08/$ - see front matter © 2008 Elsevier Inc. All rights reserved.
doi:10.1016/j.cden.2007.12.001   *dental.theclinics.com*

What is health literacy?

There are several definitions for health literacy, each of which emphasizes the availability of skills to obtain, understand, and use health information appropriately, as shown in Table 1. The World Health Organization was one of the first entities to define health literacy [1] and lead the way to further modifications [2,3]. Oral health literacy was first defined in Healthy People 2010, and is consistent with the definition for general health literacy: "The degree to which individuals have the capacity to obtain, process and understand basic health information and services needed to make appropriate oral health decisions" [3]. Inherent in all definitions is the concept that health outcomes would improve by facilitating people's access to health information and their capacity to use it effectively. In this manner health literacy skills are critical to empowering people's ability to promote and improve their health.

Table 1
Health literacy definitions compared

Definition			Keywords
WHO	"Health literacy represents the cognitive and social skills which determine the motivation and ability of individuals to gain access to, understand, and use the information in ways which promote and maintain good health."	World Health Organization	skills→ motivation and ability→ access, understand, use→ promote and maintain health
United States	"The degree to which individuals have the capacity to obtain, process and understand basic health information and services needed to make appropriate health decisions."	Ratzan & Parker [2], Healthy People 2010	Degree of capacity→ obtain, process, understand, basic information, services→ appropriate health decisions
Oral Health Literacy	"The degree to which individuals have the capacity to obtain, process and understand basic health information and services needed to make appropriate oral health decisions."	Healthy People 2010	Degree of capacity→ obtain, process, understand, basic information, services→ appropriate health decisions

Health literacy was given wide visibility with the simultaneous release of the Institute of Medicine's (IOM) report, *Health Literacy: A Prescription to End Confusion* and the Agency for Health care Research and Quality's *Literacy and Health Outcomes* [4,5]. Earlier reports highlighted aspects of the challenge facing our nation: 50% of United States adults do not read well enough to decipher a bus schedule [6]. Another IOM report, *Communicating Health: Priorities and Strategies for Progress*, emphasized that everyone has a right to science-based health information that is provided in ways that can be understood [7]. In the dental setting, the use of dental terms, such as periodontal disease, dental caries, and orthodontia can act as barriers to the understanding of most patients. The words and media we use to describe emerging science-based findings and patient information, and our health education and other print material, are our tools for effective communication. This includes diverse materials, such as newsletters, informed consent forms, insurance forms, health histories, and instructions for home care after dental procedures.

Health literacy is more than the ability to read and encompasses a number of other skills. These skills include writing, listening, numeracy or the ability to use math, and oral communication [4]. In addition, health literacy entails the ability to navigate our challenging health system and is affected by education, culture, and the context of the situation. To highlight the complexity of factors affecting health literacy, the schematic from the IOM report is shown in Fig. 1. The interactions and roles of the health care system emphasize the importance of health care providers and policy makers [4]. All health care providers are either overtly or inadvertently intimately involved in health literacy. The focus on health literacy comes at a time when our country's demographics are rapidly changing and the requirements of self-care and health services are increasing.

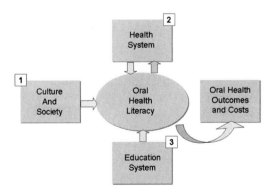

Fig. 1. Oral health literacy framework. (*Adapted from* Nielsen-Bohlman L, Panzer AM, Kindig DA. Health literacy: a prescription to end confusion. Washington, DC: National Academies Press; 2004. p. 5; with permission.)

Why is health literacy important?

The simple answer to the question of why health literacy is important is that poor or low health literacy contributes to disease, and this costs the nation and individuals a lot of money. In a recent study, it was estimated that the cost of low health literacy ranges between $106 billion to $238 billion annually [8]. This represents between 7% to 17% of all personal health care expenditures. Individuals with low health literacy have increased use of emergency care, poor control of diabetes, and are less likely to use preventive regimens and screenings than individuals with high health literacy [4]. In addition, health literacy is now recognized as an important determinant of health. Health literacy skills vary across different health topics, including diabetes, cancer, heart disease, and oral health. Health literacy is now recognized as an important determinant of health. Being able to understand health information and how to obtain services is critical to all aspects of personal health management [4,9].

Those at highest risk for low levels of health literacy include individuals 65 years of age and older, those who have less than a high school education, and those belonging to racial or ethnic minority groups [9]. According to the first national survey on health literacy, a component of the 2003 National Assessment of Adult Literacy (NAAL), Hispanic adults had lower average health literacy than adults in any other group [9]. The continuing demographic increases in racial and ethnic minorities and persons 65 years of age and older will continue to challenge our population's health literacy.

The 2003 NAAL survey also revealed that 44% of Americans responded in the intermediate level of prose literacy. Intermediate level means they can make only simple inferences and apply information from moderately dense text. For example, only one in ten United States adults is proficient in understanding health related written materials. At the other end of the phase, one in three Americans fall within either the basic level (22%) literacy or below the basic level (14%), which means they have difficulty understanding and applying health information. These survey findings highlight the mismatch between the capability of a large proportion of the United States public and the demands of the health care system [4,6,9]. Most health care information, including insurance forms, informed consent forms, patient health instruction or education materials, and hospital or clinic signs are often complex and written at reading levels far exceeding the abilities of the majority of American adults [4].

The demands of health care providers and the health care system are complex and can challenge even those who are well educated. At any given time, anyone—regardless of level of education, age, race, and ethnic characteristics—may be challenged in their interface with the United States health care system. The problem of limited health literacy is perhaps best described as a functional mismatch between the skills of the individual and the demands placed on that individual by the health care system and its providers [4]. The transmission and receipt of information depends on the capacity of both the sender and the receiver, and this capacity is affected by the setting (a dental patient being in a prone position), context (a procedure that is preventive versus one that is surgical), and format of the information delivered, among other factors.

Provider interpersonal and communication skills, and the ability of patients to understand and use the information are critical to the process. Most of us assume that our oral instructions and information are listened to, are clear, and are understood. However this assumption is not always valid, especially in health care settings where many are ill at ease and even fearful. It can be difficult to hear and understand what is being said during stressful times, and even more difficult to compose and ask relevant questions. Formal training in communication would allow us to assess the abilities of our individual patients, work with our team members to present effective and tailored oral, written, and other forms of health information.

What can you do to improve communications with your patients?

Health literacy is not just about individual patients, but also includes health care providers and other decision makers. Your first opportunity as a health care provider is to conduct a needs assessment. This includes an assessment of your office materials, an environmental scan of your facility, a review of your patient's health literacy levels, and an assessment of how you and your team can improve collaborative decision-making with your patients [10,11].

Improve the usability of health information, education and forms

Information about oral health is conveyed in a variety of forms, such as print materials, the internet, audiovisuals, and the spoken word [12–14]. All of these methods can and should be executed in plain language. Plain language is a strategy for making written and orally communicated information easier to use and understand. A plain language document, such as an educational leaflet on preventing gingivitis or a DVD demonstrating how to clean an infant's mouth, is one in which the user can find the information they need, understand it, and act appropriately on that understanding [12–14]. The key elements of a product written in plain language include having:

The most important points organized and presented first
Complex information broken down into understandable segments
Only simple language (no jargon) to define technical terms
The active voice used
Long dental or medical terms that must be used explained and spelled phonetically in parenthesis

Create a user-friendly physical environment setting for patients

Whether you see patients in a private practice setting, hospital, or a community health center you should ensure that the environment is helpful and supportive, and that it is user friendly [10,11] There are many simple but important steps that can help create this type of environment:

Have real people answer the phone, except for after hours
Provide clear directions to the office or clinic
Urge patients to write down and bring to the appointment any questions they might have about their oral health
Use only clearly written words ("x-rays" rather than "radiology") and visible signs and directions for going from one place to another
Use universal symbols where feasible and maps and color coding of various departments in large health facilities
Use health history and informed consent forms that are in plain language
Provide help in completing and or understanding all forms and educational materials

Assess your patients' level of health literacy

Several instruments have been developed to evaluate the health literacy of an individual. Most of these instruments are connected with general health and tend to be applied in research studies. Examples include the Test of Functional Health Literacy (TOFHLA), a reading comprehension instrument and its short form Short Test of/Functional Health Literacy in Adults (STOFHLA), Rapid Estimate of Adult Literacy in Medicine (REALM), a word recognition instrument, and more recently, Vital Signs, an instrument based on the use of a nutrition label [4,15]. Instruments to evaluate oral health literacy have been recently published. These instruments, REALD-30 and REALD-90, are word recognition instruments patterned after the REALM. The Test of Functional Health Literacy in Dentistry (TOFHLiD) is patterned after the TOFHLA, and consists of a reading comprehension instrument [16–18]. Generally, it is agreed that none of these instruments actually measure health literacy, rather they provide approximations of reading skills [6].

A recent assessment approach applicable to clinical settings was developed by Chew and colleagues [19] and resulted from their evaluation of a series of simple questions to identify patients with low health literacy. They compared 16 five-point Likert health literacy screening questions with the STOFHLA. Several of their questions were as effective in detecting inadequate health literacy as the STOFHLA, and they were less intrusive in a clinical setting. The validated questions are shown in Fig. 2 and can be used to identify individuals who need extra help in understanding their oral health needs and the requisite skills they need to practice for improved oral health. These four questions can be included in the health intake form or used on

1. How sure are you that you can complete medical forms correctly when you fill them out by yourself?

☐   Not at all sure

☐   A little sure

☐   Somewhat sure

☐   Quite sure

☐   Extremely sure

2. How sure are you that you can follow the written instructions on a bottle of Tylenol or aspirin?

☐   Not at all sure

☐   A little sure

☐   Somewhat sure

☐   Quite sure

☐   Extremely sure

3. How often do you have someone help you read printed materials that your health care provider gave you?

☐   Never have someone help

☐   Occasionally have someone help

☐   Sometimes have someone help

☐   Often have someone help

☐   Always have someone help

4. How often do you have problems learning about a health topic or issue because of difficulty understanding written information?

☐   Never have problems

☐   Rarely have problems

☐   Sometimes have problems

☐   Often have problems

☐   Always have problems

Fig. 2. Validated health literacy questions. (*Data from* Chew LD, Bradley KA, Boyko EJ. Brief questions to identify patients with inadequate health literacy. Fam Med 2004;36(8): 588–94.)

a separate form. If either questions 1 or 2 are in the "quite sure" or "extremely sure" category the patient will be able to understand written instructions or educational materials. If they respond in the first three categories, "not at all sure," "a little sure," or "somewhat sure" you will know that extra assistance is needed to ensure that the patient understands what is being conveyed. Similarly, regarding questions 3 and 4, if the patient responds in any of the last three options, you need to apply the recommendations in the following section.

To learn how you and your staff are doing from your patients' perspective, you may wish to use the questionnaire developed by Makoul and colleagues [20] shown in Fig. 3. This direct feedback adds another critical piece

Communication Assessment Tool

Communication with patients is a very important part of quality oral health care. We would like to know how you feel about the way your dental care provider communicated with you. Your answers are completely confidential, so please be open and honest.

1	2	3	4	5
Poor	Fair	Good	Very good	Excellent

Please use this scale to rate the way the dentist or dental hygienist communicated with you. Circle your answer for each item below.

The Dentist/Dental hygienist	Poor				Excellent	N/A
Greeted me in a way that made me feel comfortable	1	2	3	4	5	
Treated me with respect	1	2	3	4	5	
Showed interest in my ideas about my oral health	1	2	3	4	5	
Understood my main health concerns	1	2	3	4	5	
Paid attention to me (looked at me, listened carefully)	1	2	3	4	5	
Let me talk without interruptions	1	2	3	4	5	
Gave me as much information as I wanted	1	2	3	4	5	
Talked in terms I could understand	1	2	3	4	5	
Showed me how to do oral hygiene procedures	1	2	3	4	5	
Had me demonstrate how to do the oral hygiene procedures	1	2	3	4	5	
Checked to be sure I understood everything	1	2	3	4	5	
Encouraged me to ask questions	1	2	3	4	5	
Involved me in decisions as much as I wanted	1	2	3	4	5	
Discussed next steps, including any follow-up plans	1	2	3	4	5	
Showed care an concern	1	2	3	4	5	
Spent the right amount of time with me	1	2	3	4	5	

The dentist's staff

Treated me with respect	1	2	3	4	5

Fig. 3. Communication assessment tool. (*Courtesy of* Gregory Makoul, PhD, Chicago, IL. Copyright © 2004.)

of information. If for example, a patient marks a 1, 2, or 3 to any of the items, the dentist and dental team should take immediate steps to correct the situation. If several patients respond to the same item, "Treated me with respect" in the 1, 2, or 3 category, you need to assess the situation immediately. The questionnaire can be used anonymously and provide information that can be used for practice changes.

Beyond the use of assessment tools, office staff might observe cues from patients who have trouble understanding the written word. For example, if a patient takes a long time to complete a health history or informed consent form and or does not complete it, it might be that the patient cannot read well enough to know what is being asked. In this case, office staff should be trained to offer help in a noncondescending manner to complete the form. If upon receiving educational materials or an informed consent form on a given procedure the patient says, "I will take it home and read it, I forgot my glasses," this may be an indication that reading is a very difficult task for them. If a patient has skipped referrals or tests, they may not have understood the instructions or are unsure about how to proceed [4].

Build knowledge to improve healthy decision-making

There are several actions you and your staff can take to facilitate healthy decision making by your patients and to avoid miscommunication. First, ask your patients how they like to learn. Do they learn best by reading, watching a video, seeing diagrams, a verbal one-to-one exchange, or a combination of these methods? This information should be noted in their health history. Second, use patient-centered strategies to explain procedures, alternative procedures, and the potential risks of each. The following actions will help you communicate with your patients:

Listen carefully to what your patient has to say.

Slow down and use short statements. Provide information in a logical, step by step manner.

Use visual aids when appropriate.

Use the "teach back" method. This means for example, when you have explained and demonstrated to the mother of a young child how, where, and when to look for white spots in her child's mouth, ask her to explain the procedure to you and preferably have her demonstrate it to you. Similarly, when you teach a mother how to clean her child's mouth, ask her to demonstrate how to do it. Or, if you have explained how to clean around a fixed bridge, you not only explain it and demonstrate it, but also ask the patient to explain and demonstrate it to you. On subsequent visits, of course, it is essential that these skills are assessed again and instructions are reinforced. All of these activities should be documented in the patient's record. Never, ask a question that has a yes or no response, such as "do you understand?" or "did you brush your teeth this morning?" These kinds of questions will almost certainly get a nod or verbal yes. Instead, ask the patient "when did you last brush your teeth?" If patient education videos are used, personal interaction with the patient should be built into the session. Patients should be asked to do something, such as respond verbally, write, or demonstrate something in response to the instruction [4,12–14,21].

Next steps

The single most important activity to do before embarking on any health promotion activity is to formulate a plan of action. With the input gained by your needs assessment, you will be able to develop an action plan. The Appendix lists further reading you may find helpful. Your action plan should have a goal, specific actions, a timetable, and an evaluation process. For example, your goal may be to "increase capacity of office/clinic staff to

improve oral health literacy of patients by focusing on disease prevention."
Steps to be taken to address this action could include:

Making updated, evidence-based scientific information on preventive
procedures readily available to staff.

Reviewing all print materials designed for patients to determine whether
they are written in plain language. Winnow out those documents that
do not qualify. Purchase or prepare new materials.

Providing training in communication skills for staff members.

Reviewing the office environment to determine whether it encourages
active communication between patients and your team. Make adjust-
ments to the setting and appointments as appropriate.

Determining health literacy capacity of your patients and make adjust-
ments accordingly.

Once you have established your goal, action steps, and a timetable, identify the roles and responsibilities of each team member and set aside time to
review the status of your plan's progress. A team approach is necessary to
improve oral health literacy. While all members of your staff have a responsibility to ensure clear communication, as the team leader you are the role
model for clear communication.

Summary

A large part of the American public has low health literacy skills. While
these are often the very individuals who have the highest treatment needs
and little or limited public or private insurance, all individuals would benefit
from enhanced health literacy skills. The nation's health promotion and disease prevention objectives call for action to be taken to improve health literacy. Specific objectives include a focus on health literacy and call for
increasing "the proportion of persons with proficient health literacy," "decreasing the proportion of persons with below basic health literacy," and
"improving the ability of providers to communicate with their patients"
[3]. Research on oral health literacy is emerging and an agenda has been
proposed [22]. We have learned from studies that physician-patient communication and adherence to a prescribed regimen is correlated [23]. We have
learned that low oral health literacy among adult patients seeking dental
care affects their ability of patients to process and understand oral health information [24]. The American Dental Association's National Oral Health
Literacy Advisory Committee is developing recommendations and programs to support the profession in this endeavor and to address the Healthy
People 2010 objectives on this topic. Oral health literacy is the new impera-
tive for our profession, one that provides us with the opportunity to build
on the foundation of our practices and improve our communication with
our patients.

Appendix

Additional health literacy resources

Harvard School of Public Health, Department of Society, Human Development, & Health, Health Literacy Studies. A variety of resources on health literacy. Available at: healthliteracy@hsph.harvard.edu.

Communicating health: priorities and strategies for progress. This publication is an action plan for the six health communication objectives found in Healthy People 2010. Available at: http://odphp.osophs.dhhs.gov/projects/healthComm/.

Scientific and technical information: simply put. This publication will help you translate complicated scientific technical information into "living room" language. Available at: www.ced.gov/communications/resources/simpput.pdf.

A family physician's practical guide to culturally competent care. This guide includes cultural competency curriculum modules to help increase family physicians with awareness, knowledge, and skills in cultural competency. Available at: http://cccm.thinkculturalhealth.org/.

References

[1] World Health Organization. Health promotion glossary. Geneva (Switzerland): World Health Organization; 1998.

[2] Ratzan SC, Parker RM. Introduction. In: Selden CR, Zorn M, Ratzan C. et al, editors. National Library of Medicine: health literacy. Bethesda (MD): National Institutes of Health, US Department of Health and Human Services. NLM pub no. CBM 2000–1.

[3] Healthy People 2010. Available at: www.healthypeople.gov. Accessed September 15, 2007.

[4] Institute of Medicine of the National Academies. Health literacy: a prescription to end confusion. Washington, DC: National Academy Press; 2004.

[5] Berkman ND, DeWalt DA, Pignone MP, et al. Literacy and health outcomes. Evidence report/technology assessment No. 87 (Prepared by RTI International-University of North Carolina Evidence-based Practice Center under Contract No. 290-02-0016). AHRQ Publication No. 04-E007-2. Rockville (MD): L Agency for Healthcare Research and Quality; 2004.

[6] Rudd RE. Health literacy skills of U.S. adults. Am J Health Behav 2007;31(1):S8–18.

[7] Institute of Medicine of the National Academies. Speaking of health: assessing health communication strategies for diverse populations. Washington, DC: National Academy Press; 2002.

[8] University of Connecticut School of Business. News release. New report estimates cost of low health literacy between $106–$236 billion dollars annually. October 10, 2007.

[9] Kutner M, Greenberg E, Jin Y, et al. The health literacy of America's adults: results from the 2003 National Assessment of Adult Literacy (NCES 2006-483). U.S. Department of Education. Washington, DC: National Center for Education Statistics; 2006.

[10] Rudd RE, Anderson JE. The health literacy environment of hospitals and health centers. Available at: www.ncsall.net and www.hsph.harvard.edu/healthliteracy. Accessed October 1, 2007.

[11] American Medical Association Foundation. Health literacy and patient safety: help patients understand; 2007. p. 65.

[12] At the heart of plain language. Available at: www.plainlanguagenetwork.org/. Accessed August 15, 2007.

[13] Plainlanguage.gov. Available at: http://www.plainlanguage.gov/. Accessed August 15, 2007.
[14] Doak CC, Doak LG, Root JH. Teaching patients with low literacy skills. 2nd edition. Philadelphia: JB Lippincott Company; 1996.
[15] Osborn CY, Weiss BD, Davis TC, et al. Measuring adult literacy in health care: performance of the newest vital sign. Am J Health Behav 2007;31(1):S36–46.
[16] Lee JY, Rozier RG, Lee SYD, et al. Development of a word recognition instrument to test health literacy in dentistry: the REALD-30-A brief communication. J Public Health Dent 2007;67:94–8.
[17] Richman JA, Lee JY, Rozier RG, et al. Evaluation of a word recognition instrument to test health literacy in dentistry: the REALD-99. J Public Health Dent 2007;67:99–104.
[18] Gong DA, Lee JY, Rozier RG, et al. Development and testing of the test of functional health literacy in dentistry (TOFHLiD). J Public Health Dent 2007;67:105–12.
[19] Chew LD, Bradley KA, Boyko EJ. Brief questions to identify patients with inadequate health literacy. Fam Med 2004;36(8):588–94.
[20] Makoul G, Krupat E, Chang CH. Measuring patient views of physician communication skills: development and testing of the communication assessment tool. Patient Educ Couns 2007;67:333–42.
[21] Schwartzberg JG, Cowett A, VanGeest J, et al. Communication techniques for patients with low health literacy: a survey of physicians, nurses, and pharmacists. Am J Health Behav 2007;31(1):S96–104.
[22] The invisible barrier: literacy and its relationship with oral health. J Public Health Dent 2005; 65:172–84.
[23] Hall JA, Roter DL, Katz NR. Meta-analysis of correlates of provider behavior in medical encounters. Med Care 1988;26:657–75.
[24] Jones M, Lee JY, Rozier RG. Oral health literacy among adult patients seeking dental care. J Am Dent Assoc 2007;138:1199–208.

THE DENTAL
CLINICS
OF NORTH AMERICA

Dent Clin N Am 52 (2008) 345–365

Patient- and Population-Reported Outcomes in Public Health Dentistry: Oral Health-Related Quality of Life

R. Gary Rozier, DDS, MPH*,
Bhavna T. Pahel, BDS, MPH

*Department of Health Policy and Administration, School of Public Health,
1105F McGavran-Greenberg Hall, CB#7411, University of North Carolina at Chapel Hill,
Chapel Hill, NC 27599-7411, USA*

The twentieth century was noteworthy in dentistry for the many epidemiologic advances that occurred in the study of oral diseases and conditions. A largely biologic perspective to these epidemiologic studies contributed a wealth of valuable information about the burden of oral diseases, how it has changed over time, and its distribution among the population according to important demographic and social characteristics. Major advances have likewise been made in the prevention and treatment of many oral diseases, and their effects on reducing the disease burden is both observable and pronounced. For adults, the prevalence of dental caries, periodontal diseases, and tooth loss declined in the 1990s, with major improvements occurring for some conditions among black nonHispanics and Mexican Americans. Yet conditions worsened for pre-school aged children and major disparities remain in almost all disease indicators [1].

Despite their enormous contributions, these biologic assessments of disease do not provide a complete picture of the burden that oral diseases pose for society because they do not measure the full impact of disease and its treatment on well being. According to the United States Surgeon General, oral diseases and conditions can "…undermine self-image and self-esteem, discourage normal social interaction, cause other health problems, and lead to chronic stress and depression as well as incur great financial cost. They may also interfere with vital functions such as breathing, food selection, eating, swallowing, and speaking and with activities of

---

* Corresponding author.
E-mail address: gary_rozier@unc.edu (R.G. Rozier).

daily living such as work, school, and family interactions" [2]. The importance that some organizations in the United States place on the impact of
oral diseases on the overall health and well-being of Americans is illustrated by excerpts from a number of documents, displayed in Table 1
[3–8].

A person usually thinks of his or her own health more broadly than
whether they have a particular disease or not, a perspective suggested by
the often observed weak statistical relationship between a person's clinical
disease status and their perceptions of their own health [9]. At the population level, although most biologic measures of oral health status among
adults in the United States improved during the 1990s, the percentage reporting the condition of their teeth or mouth as being "excellent or very
good" declined [1]. Furthermore, major cultural and sociodemographic
shifts in North American society will continue to shape the way people think
about their oral health experiences. For example, the number of public
school students in the United States who are low-income is approaching
a majority, standing at 46% in the 2006 to 2007 school year, and already
has become a majority (54%) in the South [10]. Poverty, poor education,
and inequality not only result in poor oral health but also affect the way
in which people think about their oral health.

Patient perceptions can be particularly important in oral health where
different treatment or prevention strategies can demonstrate small differences in outcomes, where some benefits may be mostly psychologic, and
where some people might not see a particular advantage to different types
of treatment. People's perspectives of the ways in which oral diseases,
conditions, and treatments affect their symptoms, function and well being
are referred to as oral health-related quality of life (OHRQoL). OHR-
QoL is one aspect of individuals' health-related quality of life (HRQoL),
and a complete separation of OHRQoL and HRQoL is not possible because oral health is one aspect of overall health. Thus, issues related to
one's overall HRQoL are relevant to those related to OHRQoL and
vice versa.

The purpose of this article is threefold. First, it reviews the relevance of
OHRQoL to public health and its use in public health practice, particularly
for monitoring the impacts of oral diseases on quality of life at the national
level, and in public health surveillance of oral disease burdens at the state
and local levels. Second, it reviews the emerging use of OHRQoL in treatment-outcomes research and program evaluation. Finally, the authors
briefly discuss the use of QHRQoL assessments in clinical practice and arguments for expanding their use in these settings, an area virtually undevel-
oped in dentistry. This review is framed by definitions of "patient reported
outcomes" and how OHRQoL and its measurement fit within this frame of
reference [11,12]. Because of this perspective, discussed in the section titled
"Defining oral health-related quality of life," the authors do not include
several categories of patient- or population-reported outcomes, such as

Table 1
Oral health-related quality of life in policy documents in the United States

Healthy People 2010 [3]	1st of 3 overall goals: To help individuals of all ages increase life expectancy and improve their quality of life. Millions of people in the United States experience dental caries, periodontal diseases, and cleft lip and cleft palate, resulting in needless pain and suffering; difficulty in speaking, chewing, and swallowing; increased costs of care; loss of self-esteem; decreased economic productivity through lost work and school days; and, in extreme cases, death. Poor oral health and untreated oral diseases and conditions can have a significant impact on quality of life.
Surgeon General's National Call to Action to Promote Oral Health [4]	...people care about their oral health, are able to articulate the problems they face, and can devise ingenious solutions to resolve them—often through creative partnerships. Ultimately, the measure of success for any of these actions will be the degree to which individuals and communities—the people of the nation itself—gain in overall health and well-being.
The Face of a Child: Surgeon General's Workshop and Conference on Children and Oral Health [5]	Children's oral health is important to their overall health and well-being. Dental and oral disorders can have a profound impact on children. These include the effects on growth, school attendance, medical complications of untreated oral disease, and economic/social outcomes.
Association of State and Territorial Dental Directors Guidelines State and Territorial Oral Health Programs [6]	Despite the fact that safe and effective means of maintaining oral health have benefited the majority of Americans, many still experience needless pain and suffering, have oral diseases that impact their overall health and well-being, and have financial and social costs that diminish their quality of life and burden society.

(continued on next page)

Table 1 (*continued*)

| Centers of Disease Control Burden of Oral Disease Tool for Use by States [7] | More than any other body part, the face bears the stamp of individual identity. Attractiveness has an important effect on psychologic development and social relationships. Considering the importance of the mouth and teeth in verbal and nonverbal communication, diseases that disrupt their functions are likely to damage self-image and alter the ability to sustain and build social relationships. The social functions of individuals encompass a variety of roles, from intimate interpersonal contacts to participation in social or community activities, including employment. Dental disease and disorders can interfere with these social roles at any or all levels. Perhaps due to social embarrassment or functional problems, people with oral conditions may avoid conversation or laughing, smiling, or other nonverbal expressions that show their mouth and teeth. |
| National Institute of Dental and Craniofacial Research Strategic Plan [8] | Goal 7, Objective 2: Assess the social, educational and economic impact of oral, dental and craniofacial diseases, disorders, conditions, and birth defects. |

individuals' perceptions of their treatment needs or quality of their dental care. This article also takes a North American perspective for its review, particularly in the section addressing the first purpose of the paper.

Since Cohen and Jago [13] first called for the development of patient-based measures for the psycho-social impact of oral health problems, the literature dealing with "quality of life" in "oral health" has grown substantially. The growth during the current decade has been particularly rapid. A Medline search crossing these two terms yielded 618 English-language citations, beginning with the first publications in the 1970s through early November 2007. Seventy-eight percent of these publications occurred in 2000 or after, 18% in the 1990s, and less than 4% before 1990. For purposes of this paper, the authors have made no attempt to conduct a systematic review of the areas that are its focus. Consequently, unknown biases might be reflected in some of the discussions and conclusions.

Defining oral health-related quality of life

Defining oral health-related quality of life is difficult because the concept is illusive and abstract, multidimensional without clear demarcations of its different components, subjective and personal, individually dynamic, and evolving within and across population groups as culture and societal expectations change [14]. Locker [14] further concludes that anyone who tackles this task is faced with interpreting many concepts, theories, terms, operational definitions, and resulting measurement instruments that have their theoretic and empiric roots in an almost overwhelming number of publications in the medical literature. Nevertheless, several excellent articles have explored the conceptual and theoretic developments of OHRQoL and laid the foundation for the relative explosion of OHRQoL publications since 2000 [14–18].

Because of its complexity, no standard definition of OHRQoL exists and it may be unwise to pursue one, although research in the area needs sound conceptual and theoretic underpinnings. Because of the challenges in defining the term, many have turned to operational definitions in which possible domains are simply listed, sometimes linked to conceptual models, such as that of the World Health Organization (WHO) model of health [19]. For example, OHRQoL was defined in the Surgeon General's Report on Oral Health as a "...multidimensional construct that reflects (among other things) people's comfort when eating, sleeping, and engaging in social interaction; their self-esteem; and their satisfaction with respect to their oral health" [2]. The most widely used OHRQoL instrument, the Oral Health Impact Profile (OHIP), is based on Locker's adaptation of the WHO model, in which impacts of disease are categorized in a hierarchy ranging from symptoms primarily internal to the individual (represented in the dimension of functional limitation) to handicaps that affect social roles, such as work [20]. The domains in the OHIP include functional limitation (eg, difficulty chewing), physical pain (eg, sensitivity of teeth), psychologic discomfort (eg, self-consciousness), physical disability (eg, changes to diet), psychologic disability (eg, reduced ability to concentrate), social disability (eg, avoiding social interaction), and handicap (eg, being unable to work productively).

While no consensus definition exists for OHRQoL, experts agree about a number of its characteristics. Points of agreement from the perspective of two cancer researchers were recently reviewed in a text devoted entirely to OHRQoL [21]. They concluded that HRQoL includes: (1) a perception of one's life circumstances; (2) components that are both affective (ie, perceived pleasantness or unpleasantness of a situation) and cognitive (ie, appraisals, thoughts, and perceived satisfaction with the situation); (3) positive and negative aspects of an experience; (4) multiple, overlapping, and related domains of functioning, as reflected in the definition provided in the Surgeon General's Report on Oral Health; and (5) changes in individuals' perceptions of HRQoL over time.

Patient- and population-reported outcomes and OHRQoL

Because OHRQoL represents a personal experience and, therefore, it most appropriately is reported by individuals themselves, confusion can exist about which self-reported oral health outcomes might qualify as OHRQoL measures. Self-reported health or treatment outcome measures can vary in complexity from a single-item question about some single concept (eg, presence or absence of pain or satisfaction with a particular type of treatment) to multi-item instruments measuring several domains of health status or treatment outcomes (eg, single scales measuring a specific functional outcome, such as chewing ability, or multidimensional scales, such as the OHIP instrument with its multiple domains and related items). The anatomic and physiologic complexity of the oral cavity, the many different diseases affecting this area of the body and the numerous available treatments for them, and the many resulting symptoms and functional outcomes resulting from both diseases and treatment can result in a particularly broad array of self-reported outcomes. Some practical guidance about OHRQoL is therefore needed in any review of its application. For this guidance the authors turn to clinical trials research, particularly cancer intervention trials.

The large number of self-reported health outcomes being used in intervention clinical trials are now being referred to as "patient-reported outcomes" (PRO) [11,12]. In a recent draft guidance for industry to use in product-labeling claims, the Food and Drug Administration defined a PRO measurement as "...any aspect of a patient's health status that comes directly from the patient (ie, without the interpretation of the patient's responses by a physician or anyone else)" and may include reports of disease symptoms, treatment adverse effects, functional status, or overall well being [22].

A work group on measurement of cancer outcomes at the National Cancer Institute (NCI), after review of hundreds of applications of HRQoL, concluded that the features of HRQoL measures that distinguish them from PRO measures are that they are not only patient reported, but involve the patient's subjective assessment or evaluation of important aspects of his or her well being [23]. The implication of this distinction provided by the NCI work group is that all HRQoL measures can be classified as PRO measures, but there are PRO measures that have little or no evaluation component and, thus, would not quality as HRQoL measures. For example, the report of presence or absence of pain by someone would not quality as a HRQoL measure according to the NCI work group recommendations unless it included a personal assessment of its severity, bother, or other impact on some aspect of well being. Specifically, the NCI work group defined a HRQoL measure to include patient assessments of symptom impact, functional status, or global well-being.

The authors use these distinguishing characteristics of HRQoL provided by the NCI work group and others to guide this review of applications of

OHRQoL in public health dentistry. As noted in the introduction, some PRO measures, such as satisfaction with treatment or the process of dental care itself, are not included in this article. The authors also extend the use of this term, which has its origins primarily in the clinical trials literature to public health, and thus refer to "population-" reported outcomes when discussing population-based surveys and other population-based OHRQoL applications. Use of the term "patient-" reported outcomes is limited to applications in clinical settings.

Application of OHRQoL in public health practice

The importance of oral health in people's quality of life is a well ingrained, but to date a largely implied perspective, in the philosophy, goals, and strategies for dental public health practice (see Table 1). The three core functions of public health practice necessary for population health, articulated by the Institute of Medicine (IOM) report on the future of public health [24] and the associated 14 essential dental public health services related to these that were provided by the Association of State and Territorial Dental Directors (ASTDD) [6], are designed to identify and monitor oral health problems in populations and ensure that effective polices and programs are in place to help alleviate these problems. OHRQoL is at the core of the framework and definition for public health practice provided by the IOM and ASTDD documents.

Yet, attention to this aspect of oral health status remains largely at the conceptual level, with less attention having been given to its application to dental public health activities, such as the measurement of OHRQoL in state and local surveillance and population-based surveys, population screening programs to identify those needing referral and treatment, or the evaluation of how the implementation of public health programs affects OHRQoL, a point to be discussed in this article. At present, no data collection mechanism or process is in place in the United States to comprehensively monitor the national burden of oral diseases from the perspective of OHRQoL. This deficit is particularly important because one of the two Healthy People 2010 goals for the nation is to improve quality of life [3]. The next two sections review use of OHRQoL measures in periodic national surveys and ongoing surveillance of oral health.

Periodic national surveys

National surveys of OHRQoL in the United States have been limited largely to single-item questions on perceived oral health status or treatment needs, while a few other countries, such as Australia [25] and the United Kingdom [26–28], have included in their national, cross-sectional surveys a larger number of impacts, such as pain, problems with chewing or talking, feeling self-conscious or embarrassed, and becoming less cheerful or irritable because of oral health problems. The OHRQoL measure most frequently used in the United States is to ask the individual to rate his or her oral health on a scale from "excellent" to "poor." These ratings require that individuals engage in an evaluation of their oral health status that effectively aggregates across whatever dimensions of health are important to them. Research suggests that adults' ratings of their own oral health and parents' ratings of their children's oral health are influenced by a combination of factors, such as presence or absence of disease, physical functioning, psychologic discomfort, health behaviors, and self-ratings of general health [29–32].

The percentage of adults or parents of children in the United States reporting the condition of their own teeth and mouth or that of their children to be "poor or fair" is displayed by age in Fig. 1. According to the National Survey of Children's Health, about 10% of parents rated their children's oral health as fair or poor [33]. The percentage of adults reporting their own oral health as fair or poor was dramatically larger than for children, but varied only slightly by age group from 36.3% to 42.5% [1]. Some differences in the estimates between children and adults can be attributed to surrogate reporting by the parent for the child and differences in how the questions were asked, but for adults in particular, oral conditions have a large impact on well being.

Major disparities in perceived oral health status also are apparent from national surveys in the United States (Table 2). The most disadvantaged groups, as measured by education or poverty status, are almost twice as likely to report fair or poor oral health as the most advantaged groups

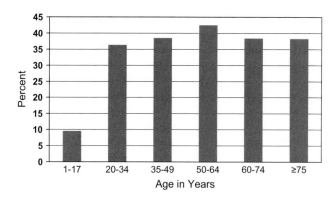

Fig. 1. Percent of subjects reporting fair or poor oral health by age, United States, 1999–2004. (*Data from* U.S. Department of Health and Human Services, Health Resources and Services Administration, Maternal and Child Health Bureau. The oral health of children: a portrait of the nation. The National Survey of Children's Health 2003. Rockville (MD): U.S. Department of Health and Human Services; 2005, for age range 1–17 and from the year 2003; and Dye BA, Tan S, Smith V, et al. Trends in oral health status: United States, 1988–1994 and 1999–2004. National Center for Health Statistics. Vital Health Stat 11 2007;248:1–92; for remaining age ranges shown.)

Table 2
Percentage of adults who perceived the condition of their teeth or mouth as fair or poor, by age group, United States, 1999–2004

Characteristic	Age	
	20–64 years	65 years and older
Race and ethnicity		
White, non-Hispanic	33.9%	34.6%
Black, non-Hispanic	50.2%	61.2%
Mexican American	57.7%	66.9%
Poverty status		
Less than 100% FPL	59.9%	67.8%
100%–199% FPL	57.7%	49.0%
Greater than 200% FPL	30.3%	30.3%
Education		
Less than high school	62.3%	55.5%
High school	47.8%	36.3%
More than high school	28.2%	30.3%
Overall	38.8%	38.3%

Abbreviation: FPL, Federal Poverty Level.

Data from Dye BA, Tan S, Smith V, et al. Trends in oral health status: United States, 1988–1994 and 1999–2004. National Center for Health Statistics. Vital Health Stat 11 2007;248:1–92.

[1]. For example, 62% of adults who did not graduate from high school report fair or poor oral health status, compared with 28% who had some education beyond high school. When combined with societal measures of impact, such as days lost from school or work, oral conditions have substantial importance [34].

Single-item, impact specific questions, such as the impact of dental problems on chewing, can be helpful in determining the major dimensions through which dental problems affect well being. The 2003 National Children's Dental Health Survey in the United Kingdom asked parents to consider whether their children had experienced any problems in the previous 12 months as a result of the condition of their teeth and gums [28]. Most parents did not think that their children had been affected by an oral condition. However, from 22% to 34% of parents of 5- to 15-year-old children, depending on age, reported some type of problem occasionally or more often during the 12 months preceding the interview. The most common problem was pain (16% to 26%), followed by being embarrassed, self-conscious or worried (4% to 10%), problems with chewing or talking (5% to 7%), having to stop playing a musical instrument (4% to 7%), and becoming less cheerful or more irritable (4% to 6%). Impacts on social functioning or general health affected 2% or less of children.

On the other hand, most adults (73%) in Britain report that oral health does affect their QoL, with most of the impact being positive [26]. Negative impacts were more likely to be reported for the physical domain (eg, 9% reported a bad effect for eating) than for the social (eg, 3% for social life) or psychologic (eg, 3% mood) domains. More than 17% of Australians reported avoiding some foods because of problems with their teeth, mouth or dentures in a 2004 to 2006 national survey of adults [25].

At least 17 dental multi-item questionnaires have been developed to measure the negative impacts of disease and ill health in adults [35,36]. A small number of multi-item instruments that have been developed only recently to measure OHRQoL among children can be added to the list of adult instruments [37]. These multi-item questionnaires are helpful in studying determinants or risks for OHRQoL, particularly when OHRQoL impacts are summarized as a scale, and the findings can be valuable to those planning community-based intervention programs. These scales, with their varying domains, provide methodologic advantages in the analysis of determinants of OHRQoL because they show more variation and responsiveness than do single-item questions. Furthermore, they can more explicitly and accurately measure the domains that are considered important in conceptual models of QoL. A major disadvantage of these instruments is their large number of questions, in some cases more than 70, which limits their use to epidemiologic or clinical studies where OHRQoL outcomes are a major focus.

Nevertheless, a number of large, cross-sectional epidemiologic studies have been done in the United States and other countries that have allowed exploration of correlations or predictors of OHRQoL through sophisticated analytic techniques. These studies, conducted mostly in older adults, are helpful in examining determinants of OHRQoL and how impacts vary by important social characteristics of populations. Slade [38] has reviewed findings from these types of studies and concluded that the factors associated with poorer OHRQoL are "fewer teeth, more diseased teeth, other untreated dental disease, unmet treatment needs, episodic dental visits to treat dental problems and lower socioeconomic status." He also concludes that "nonwhite respondents (in the United States) generally have poorer OHRQoL compared with white respondents."

Another important question for dental public health practice is whether some oral diseases or conditions present particularly strong and negative impacts on well being, and therefore should receive special consideration in planning dental public health programs. It appears that dentofacial problems, such as cleft lip or palate, skeletal and dental mal-alignments, oral and pharyngeal cancers, temporo-mandibular joint dysfunctions, salivary gland dysfunctions resulting from conditions such as Sjogren's syndrome, and severe early childhood caries can result in particularly strong impacts on QoL [2].

Public health surveillance

The National Oral Health Surveillance System (NOHSS), designed to provide more frequent and more local data on the burden of oral diseases in the United States than the national periodic surveys discussed in the previous section, does not include any OHRQoL measures. Rather, it includes eight indicators for oral disease (oral and pharyngeal cancer, dental caries experience, untreated dental caries, complete tooth loss), use of the oral health care delivery system (dental visits, teeth cleaning, dental sealants), and the status of community water fluoridation [39]. The NOHSS relies primarily on available national surveys that can provide state-level estimates, as well as clinical information collected by state or local programs according to a standard protocol. The national survey, known as the Behavioral Risk Factor and Surveillance System (BFRSS), which provides several indicators (visits, cleaning, tooth loss), does not include any patient- or population-reported outcomes for oral health status.

Very few states have their own surveillance system for the impact of oral diseases and conditions on well being. Colorado and North Carolina have implemented annual surveys that include OHRQoL indicators for children, specifically, a single question on global oral health status [40,41]. In those states, parents of school-aged children or younger who are sampled as part of the BRFSS, which only includes information about adults, are included in a follow-up survey about their children's health. The reported OHRQoL measure on these state surveys is a single question on global oral health status [40,41]. The results are similar to the national average, with 9.1% and 7.8% of parents in Colorado and North Carolina, respectively, reporting that their children's oral health is fair or poor. Major disparities in parents' perceived condition of children's teeth also are apparent, with, for example, 20.7% of Hispanic parents in North Carolina reporting fair or poor oral health status for their children, compared with 6.5% of other ethnic groups. The growing racial and ethnic diversity of the United States population also is, of course, an important consideration in planning dental public health programs. Such planning should entail consideration not only of cultural differences in perceptions of treatment needs, but also how these diverse groups interpret and perceive their OHRQoL.

Lastly, public health research in recent years has been enriched by concepts and ideas from the life course framework that emphasize the role of events that occur early in life on population health outcomes later in life. This approach should be extended to include effects on OHRQoL. For example, a recent study from Brazil reported that the incidence of enamel defects is associated with life course events, such as early malnutrition and pre- and postnatal infections among a cohort of children from low-income families [42]. Although the investigators did not measure changes in quality of life, their results point to the importance of considering OHRQoL as an outcome measure in longitudinal population-based studies.

OHRQoL outcomes from individual- and population-targeted interventions

An emerging area of interest in OHRQoL is its application to outcomes research and the use of what is learned from these studies by clinicians, managers, and policymakers in decision making. Treatment-outcomes research, which emerged in the 1980s from the recognition that large geographic variation in treatments exist but with similar outcomes, seeks to understand the end results of health care interventions from the perspective of patients and what is important to them. By linking the care people get to the outcomes they experience, outcomes research has become a key to developing better ways to monitor and improve the quality of health care. As a part of this movement, traditional biomedical end-points of clinical trials have been expanded to include measures of how people function and their experiences with care [43,44]. By extension to public health practice, treatment-outcomes research includes program evaluation.

OHRQoL and clinical treatment outcomes

As might be expected, most clinical trials in which patients' perspectives of treatment outcomes are considered have been conducted for dental conditions that potentially can have substantial negative impacts on people's physical, psychologic, and social functioning. These studies also usually include treatments with relatively equal or unknown effectiveness, have different costs, and result in outcomes not always satisfactory to the patient.

A large number of outcome studies have been done for prosthodontic treatment of tooth loss. A systematic review of the influence of implant and conventional prostheses on satisfaction and quality of life identified 114 such studies [45,46]. Most of these used single-item measures of patient satisfaction or selected OHRQoL domains to measure outcomes. Seventeen of the studies were classified as randomized controlled trials, all of which evaluated outcomes of implant therapy, mostly for the treatment of edentulous patients. The conclusion from this systematic review was that the OHRQoL of patients benefits from the use of dental implants to support mandibular prostheses. Investigators also concluded that few studies provided strong evidence of effect on OHRQoL, with additional research needed, particularly of treatments for the partially edentulous patient and single crowns.

Other dental treatments are not well studied. OHRQoL has been reported as an outcome, for example, in the use of splints in patients with temporomandibular disorders [47], surgery for periodontal disease [48], mobile dental services for frail residents in adult day care health centers [49], and surgery for head and neck cancers [50]. The systematic review by the Cochrane Collaboration on the effectiveness of screening for oral cancer found only one study, and it did not include an assessment of QoL or harms from the screening [51]. The Cochrane systematic review of surgical treatments for head and neck cancers concluded that few trials report on adverse events associated with treatment or subsequent quality of life [50].

In general, those who have reviewed treatment-outcome studies in dentistry have concluded that the literature does not provide strong evidence of effects on OHRQoL because of the small number of studies for any one treatment and their weak experimental designs [46,50]. Treatment-outcomes research in dentistry must be considered as being in the initial formative stages, and thus provides many opportunities for health services research.

OHRQoL and program evaluation

Program evaluation is a core function in dental public health practice and highly valued for its contributions [24]. But to date, this function of public health has largely been underfunded and has concentrated primarily on process measures, such as the number of people served or, less frequently, on biodental or dental services outcomes, such as the number of cavities prevented or treatments averted. Economic evaluations also have played an important role in dental public health decision making because of the predominate use of public funds to support community-based interventions, such as community water fluoridation. Population-centered OHRQoL outcome measures can compliment and even provide necessary information for decision making in dental public health, but their use is in the formative stages of development [52].

The evaluation of water fluoridation serves as a case in point. More than 150 million people in the United States are exposed to this public health intervention and countless people have been spared the negative consequences of dental caries as a result [53]. It always has been known that this intervention carries with it a single risk of enamel fluorosis for a portion of the population. Decisions about its implementation thus must consider this balance between its beneficial effect on preventing dental caries and its risk of causing fluorosis, a condition mostly of esthetic concern. Historically, programmatic decisions about water fluoridation have been heavily influenced by the high prevalence of disease and ready population penetration that water fluoridation offers, particularly for reaching disadvantaged populations who have limited access to other preventive dental services. However, the risk-benefit relationship changed in the 1980s because of the dramatic declines in the prevalence and severity of dental caries and observed increases in the prevalence and severity of enamel fluorosis [53–57].

The amount and severity of fluorosis occurring with water fluoridation have long been considered of little cosmetic importance from the perspective of dental professionals [57]. Yet, only recently has the public's perceptions of enamel fluorosis been assessed [58–69]. Results of these studies consistently show that people can have esthetic concerns about teeth, and that fluorosis can be a primary factor in their dissatisfaction, particularly in its more severe forms. They generally express dissatisfaction when fluoride-induced opacities affect the entire visible tooth surface. Because enamel fluorosis is the only side effect from water fluoridation and this condition is of esthetic concern only, the public's perceptions of the effects of fluorosis on appearances are important in considering the risks and benefits of this public health intervention.

Important research recently completed by Do and Spencer [70,71] at the Australian Research Center for Population Oral Health, has considered the risk-benefit relationship for water fluoridation using both a biologic perspective and a population perspective. As expected based on previous studies, they found an association between water fluoridation exposure and both caries and fluorosis among the same children. But they also found that the population impact of water fluoridation differed for the two conditions. They estimated that 63 out of every 1,000 South Australian children had fluorosis because of water fluoridation, compared with 111 children who were prevented from having caries at 6 years of age. It is clear that more cases of disease were prevented by water fluoridation in these children than were cases of fluorosis caused by water fluoridation.

Yet this clinical perspective does not consider child or parent perspectives about benefits or side effects of water fluoridation—the potential positive impacts of caries prevention and the potential negative impacts of dental fluorosis—on OHRQoL. Here is where the research by Do and Spencer provides a major advance in our understanding of the risks and benefits of water fluoridation and demonstrates the value of OHRQoL in the evaluation of dental public health programs.

Do and Spencer used both global ratings of oral health status and multi-item OHRQoL scales (Parent-Caregiver and Child Perceptions Questionnaires developed by Jokovic and colleagues [72–74]) to determine the impact of caries and fluorosis on children and parents. Among this child population, about 30% had some degree of fluorosis and about half had some experience with dental caries. An overall interpretation of both parents' global ratings of their children's oral health status and the multi-item scales suggests that caries experience in children has a negative effect on parents' ratings of OHRQoL, particularly in the domain of oral symptoms, and that mild fluorosis has a positive effect on OHRQoL. These relationships derived from the bivariate analyses are displayed in Fig. 2. The mean OHRQoL scores are lower for fluorosis scores of "1" and "2" than for scores of "0" or "3," indicating fewer negative impacts on OHRQoL with mild fluorosis. Conversely, mean OHRQoL scores increase with each category of increasing dental caries, indicating a greater number of negative impacts on OHRQoL with increasing severity of caries. These results suggest that at a population level, water fluoridation improves OHRQoL because it lessens the negative impacts from both dental caries and tooth appearance.

Assessing OHRQoL in clinical practice

Clinicians such as physicians, dentists, and nurses informally assess OHRQoL in most patient encounters with questions like: "Does the tooth keep you awake at night?" "Does the pain in your jaw keep you from eating the things you like?" or "Are you satisfied with the appearance of your new

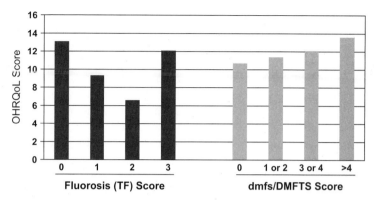

Fig. 2. Parents' oral health-related quality of life ratings by severity of enamel fluorosis and dental caries in their children. OHRQoL score: Sum of 5-point Likert scale for the Parent-Caregiver and Child Perceptions Questionnaires, rated from 0 = "never" to 4 = "very often." TF: Thylstrup & Fejerskov modified Fluorosis Index (1988) ranging from 0 = "normal" to 3 = "opacity involving many parts of surface" [72–74]. (*Data from* Do LG, Spencer AJ. Oral health-related quality of life of children by dental caries and fluorosis experience. J Public Health Dent 2007;67:132–9.)

dentures, and have any of your friends noticed them?" More formal assessments of patients' OHRQoL are rare in the clinical practice of medicine or dentistry, but strong arguments for their use have been put forward for both disciplines [12,75–77].

Among the arguments made for more formal measures of the impact of illnesses and treatments on patients' QoL in clinical care are that they can:

- Improve communication and shared decision making between patients and providers
- Record the health status of patients entering treatment and identify who will benefit because they have treatable problems
- Determine the degree and sources of the patient's decreased ability to function
- Distinguish among types of problems, including physical, emotional and social
- Detect adverse outcomes from treatment
- Monitor the effects of disease progression and response to treatment
- Predict the course of disease, treatment needs and outcomes of care

At present, it is difficult to provide scientific evidence to support any of these reasons to use OHRQoL assessments in patient dental care. None of the current instruments were designed specifically for these purposes nor have they been tested in these clinical settings to any large extent.

Use of the short version of the OHIP in a sample of patients in six dental practices in Scotland, as part of a longitudinal observational study, suggests that this measure has acceptable psychometric properties in this setting and is responsive to changes in third molar symptoms [78]. Research is needed on the application of OHRQoL to the care of dental patients, beginning with very fundamental research related to the performance of OHRQoL scales in clinical dental care settings, particularly their responsiveness to changes in clinical symptoms and treatment outcomes [9,17]. One area of growing interest is in the use of OHRQoL measures to better understand clinically important differences in oral disease conditions from the patient's perspective (known as the "minimally important clinical difference" in patient-reported outcomes), which in turn can be used to inform patient-centered oral health care [79].

The public health workforce has an important role in providing clinical care to underserved populations through community-based programs, so the previous comments about the use of OHRQoL in clinical practice apply to public health clinics as well. At a broader level, public health also has an important responsibility to monitor the quality of clinical care that the public is receiving in all clinical settings, not just public health, particularly in those delivery systems involving large, defined patient populations such as the military, Medicaid, or the incarcerated. Beyond monitoring responsibilities, public health agencies often are charged with the responsibility to develop and promote interventions and policies that will improve the quality of care. Considerations of the effects of clinical prevention and treatment services on OHRQoL are closely tied to concerns about the quality of care and the movement to document and improve quality.

Interest in measuring the quality of dental care has led to the development of new measures for clinical effectiveness of dental care and satisfaction of consumers, mostly for use at the insurance-plan level [80,81]. Patient surveys have been developed to measure discrete features of dental plan performance, the dental care setting, and the behaviors of practitioners [82–84]. California is actively involved in satisfaction surveys of members of its public insurance dental programs [82,83]. In addition, the United States military is engaged in developing a method to benchmark the performance of its dental health care system using OHRQoL information from its soldiers and family members [84]. The activities in California and the United States military include a global measure of OHRQoL in its surveys.

Given the potential benefits to clinical practice, management of delivery systems, and policy decision making about the delivery of dental care, consideration should be given to experimenting in clinical settings with specific patient-reported outcomes related to the impact of dental care on QoL. This area of dental public health research and development will be faced with a number of challenges, such as resource constraints in collecting, assembling, and constructing reports, not unlike problems faced for other clinical information systems. However, ongoing attempts to benchmark and improve the quality of clinical care for patients will provide excellent opportunities to include OHRQoL outcomes in these settings.

Summary

Several conclusions are evident from this review of OHRQoL and public health dentistry. First, large-scale population surveys in the United States and other countries usually have included only single-question assessments of OHRQoL, most often a global health rating. Rarely have assessments included multiple-item questionnaires. Surveys have been limited mostly to population-based or clinic-based surveys done for specific study purposes. The National Oral Health Surveillance System does not include any OHRQoL indicators, and to the authors' knowledge, few states have included any in their surveillance systems for children or adults.

Nevertheless, sufficient evidence exists to conclude that oral diseases and their treatment place a large burden on society and its well being. A substantial percentage of the population rates their oral health badly, and major disparities are evident similar to those that appear with access to dental health services, use of care, or biologic indicators. Dental disease causes pain and loss of physical and social function, including compromised ability to chew and achieve proper nutrition, and accomplish daily activities such as attending school or work.

Second, the use of OHRQoL in treatment or community intervention outcomes studies is an emerging area of health services research and public health evaluation, with QoL only beginning to be considered as an important secondary outcome, if not primary outcome, for those conditions that can be prevented or treated with different methods and costs. Results of completed outcome studies show that dental treatments and community interventions can improve OHRQoL. However, clinical research has not been extended much beyond prosthodontics, and methodologic research is needed to ensure that impacts of treatment on areas of QoL can be measured accurately and detect meaningful differences. Few studies of the impact of population-based interventions on OHRQoL have been conducted, but one study on water fluoridation demonstrates positive impacts and serves as an excellent example of the importance of this emerging area of program evaluation in public health.

Finally, virtually no work has been done to investigate applications of OHRQoL in assessing the standard of clinical care for patients. Assessments of patients' perspectives as part of their clinical care have the potential to improve the quality of that care, patient satisfaction, and its outcomes. These applications can also be considered an important aspect of public health dentistry's responsibility to ensure the quality of patient care. The intersection of movements in quality and patient-centered care provide the opportunity for public health research and potential inclusion of measures of OHRQoL in patients' assessments of the care they receive in dental offices.

References

[1] Dye BA, Tan S, Smith V, et al. Trends in oral health status: United States, 1988–1994 and 1999–2004. National Center for Health Statistics. Vital Health Stat 11 2007;248:1–92.

[2] U.S. Department of Health and Human Services. Oral health in America: a report of the Surgeon General. Rockville (MD): U.S. Department of Health and Human Services, National Institute of Dental and Craniofacial Research, National Institutes of Health; 2000.

[3] U.S. Department of Health and Human Services. Healthy People 2010. vols. 2. 2nd edition. Washington, DC: U.S. Government Printing Office; 2000.

[4] U.S. Department of Health and Human Services. A National Call to Action to Promote Oral Health. Rockville (MD): U.S. Department of Health and Human Services, Public Health Service, Centers for Disease Control and Prevention, National Institutes of Health, National Institute of Dental and Craniofacial Research; 2003, NIH Publication No. 03-5303.

[5] National Institute of Dental and Craniofacial Research. Proceedings of the face of a child: Surgeon General's 2000 Conference on Children and Oral Health. Bethesda (MD): U.S. Department of Health and Human Services; 2000. Available at: http://www.nidcr.nih.gov/sgr/children/children.htm. Accessed November 1, 2007.

[6] Association of State and Territorial Dental Directors. Guidelines for state and territorial oral health programs; 2007. Available at: http://www.astdd.org/docs/ASTDDGuidelines.pdf. Accessed November 17, 2005.

[7] Centers for Disease Control and Prevention. The burden of oral disease: tool for creating state documents. Atlanta (GA): U.S. Department of Health and Human Services; 2005. Available at: http://www.cdc.gov/oralhealth/library/burdenbook/. Accessed November 17, 2005.

[8] National Institute of Dental and Craniofacial Research. NIDCR strategic plan. The burden of oral diseases. National Institutes of Health, National Institute of Dental and Craniofacial Research; 2003. Available at: http://www.nidcr.nih.gov/AboutNIDCR/StrategicPlan/default.htm. Accessed November 1, 2007.

[9] Locker D, Jokovic A. Using subjective oral health status indicators to screen for dental care in older adults. Community Dent Oral Epidemiol 1996;24:398–402.

[10] Suitts S. A new majority: low income students in the South's public schools. Southern Education Foundation; 2007. Available at: http://www.southerneducation.org/. Accessed November 2, 2007.

[11] Acquadro C, Berzon R, Dubois D, et al. Incorporating the patient's perspective into drug development and communication: an ad hoc task force report of the Patient-Reported Outcomes (PRO) Harmonization Group meeting at the Food and Drug Administration, February 16, 2001. Value Health 2003;6:522–31.

[12] Lipscomb J, Gotay CC, Snyder CF. Patient-reported outcomes in cancer: a review of recent research and policy initiatives. CA Cancer J Clin 2007;57:278–300.

[13] Cohen LK, Jago JD. Toward formulation of socio-dental indicators. Int J Health Serv 1976; 6:681–98.

[14] Locker D. Concepts of oral health, disease and the quality of life. In: Slade GD, editor. Measuring oral health and quality of life. Chapel Hill (NC): University of North Carolina Dental Ecology; 1997. p. 12–23.

[15] Ferrans CE. Definitions and conceptual models of quality of life. In: Lipscomb J, Gotay CC, Snyder C, editors. Outcomes assessment in cancer: measures, methods, and applications. Cambridge (UK): Cambridge University Press; 2005. p. 14–30.

[16] Locker D. Measuring oral health: a conceptual framework. Community Dent Health 1988;5: 5–13.

[17] Reisine S, Locker D. Social, psychological and economic impacts of oral conditions and treatments. In: Cohen LK, Gift HC, editors. Disease prevention and oral health promotion. 1st edition. Copenhagen (Denmark): Munksgaard; 1995. p. 33–72.

[18] Wilson IB, Cleary PD. Linking clinical variables with health-related quality of life: a conceptual model of patient outcomes. JAMA 1995;273:59–65.

[19] World Health Organization. International classification of impairments, disabilities and handicaps: a manual of classification. Geneva (Switzerland): World Health Organization; 1980.

[20] Slade GD, Spencer AJ. Development and evaluation of the oral health impact profile. Community Dent Health 1994;11:3–11.

[21] Cimprich B, Paterson AG. Health-related quality of life: conceptual issues and research applications [chapter 5]. Inglehart MR, Bagramian RA, editors. Oral health-related quality of life. Chicago: Quintessence Publishing Co, Inc; 2002. p. 47–53.

[22] U.S. Department of Health and Human Services, Food and Drug Administration, Center for Drug Evaluation and Research (CDER), Center for Biologics Evaluation and Research (CBER), Center for Devices and Radiological Health (CDRH). Guidance for industry-patient-reported outcome measures: use in medical product development to support labeling claims. Available at: http://www.fda.gov/cber/gdlns/prolbl.pdf. Accessed November 12, 2007.

[23] Lipscomb J, Gotay CC, Snyer C. Introduction to outcomes assessment in cancer. In: Lipscomb J, Gotay CC, Snyder C, editors. Outcomes assessment in cancer: measures, methods, and applications. Cambridge (UK): Cambridge University Press; 2005. p. 1–14.

[24] Institute of Medicine. The future of public health. Washington, DC: National Academy Press; 1988.

[25] Slade GD, Spencer AJ, Roberts-Thomson KF. Australia's dental generations. The National Survey of Adult Oral Health 2004–06. Canberra: Australian Institute of Health and Welfare (Dental Statistics and Research Series No. 34); 2007, AIHW cat. No. DEN 165.

[26] McGrath C, Bedi R. Measuring the impact of oral health on quality of life in Britain using OHQoL-UK(W). J Public Health Dent 2003;63:73–7.

[27] Kelly M, Steele J, Nuttall N, et al. Adult dental health survey: oral health in the United Kingdom 1998. London: The Stationary Office; 2000.

[28] Lader D, Chadwick B, Chestnutt I, et al. Children's dental health in the United Kingdom, 2003. London: Office of National Statistics; 2005.

[29] Gift HC, Atchison KA, Drury TF. Perceptions of the natural dentition in the context of multiple variables. J Dent Res 1998;77:1529–38.

[30] Locker D, Wexler E, Jokovic A. What do older adults' global self-ratings of oral health measure? J Public Health Dent 2005;65:146–52.

[31] Talekar BS, Rozier RG, Slade GD, et al. Parental perceptions of their preschool-aged children's oral health. J Am Dent Assoc 2005;136:364–72.

[32] Weyant RJ, Manz M, Corby P, et al. Factors associated with parents' and adolescents' perceptions of oral health and need for dental treatment. Community Dent Oral Epidemiol 2007;35:321–30.

[33] U.S. Department of Health and Human Services, Health Resources and Services Administration, Maternal and Child Health Bureau. The oral health of children: a portrait of the nation. The National Survey of Children's Health 2003. Rockville (MD): U.S. Department of Health and Human Services; 2005.

[34] Gift HC. Research directions in oral health promotion for older adults. J Dent Educ 1992;56: 626–31.

[35] Slade GD, editor. Measuring oral health and quality of life. Chapel Hill (NC): University of North Carolina Dental Ecology; 1997. p. 12–23.

[36] Brondani MA, MacEntee JI. The concept of validity in sociodental indicators and oral health-related quality-of-life measures. Community Dent Oral Epidemiol 2007;35:472–8.

[37] Slade GD, Resine ST. The Child Oral Health Impact Profile: current status and future directions. Community Dent Oral Epidemiol 2007;35(Suppl 1):50–3.

[38] Slade GD. Assessment of oral health-related quality of life [chapter 4]. Inglehart MR, Bagramian RA, editors. Oral health-related quality of life. Chicago: Quintessence Publishing Co, Inc; 2002. p. 29–46.

[39] Beltrán-Aguilar ED, Malvitz DM, Lockwood SA, et al. Oral health surveillance: past, present, and future challenges. J Public Health Dent 2003;63:141–9.

[40] Colorado Department of Public Health and Environment. Colorado child health survey results, 2006. Denver (CO): Health Statistics; 2006. Available at: http://www.cdphe.state.co.us/hs/yrbs/ChildHealthDental2.html. Accessed November 21, 2007.

[41] NC Department of Health and Human Services. 2006 North Carolina statewide CHAMP survey. Raleigh (NC): State Center for Health Statistics; 2006. Available at: http://www.schs.state.nc.us/SCHS/champ/2006/k16q02.html. Accessed November 21, 2007.

[42] Chaves AM, Rosenblatt A, Oliveira OF. Enamel defects and its relation to life course events in primary dentition of Brazilian children: a longitudinal study. Community Dent Health 2007;24:31–6.

[43] Clancy CM, Eisenberg JM. Outcomes research: measuring the end results of health care. Science 1998;282:245–6.

[44] Gerszten PC. Outcomes research: a review. Neurosurgery 1998;43:1146–55.

[45] Strassburger C, Heydecke G, Kerschbaum T. Influence of prosthetic and implant therapy on satisfaction and quality of life: a systematic literature review. Part 1: Characteristics of the studies. Int J Prosthodont 2004;17:83–93.

[46] Strassburger C, Heydecke G, Kerschbaum T. Influence of implant and conventional prostheses on satisfaction and quality of life: a literature review. Part 2: Qualitative analysis and evaluation of the studies. Int J Prosthodont 2006;19:229–48.

[47] Dao TT, Lavigne GJ, Charbonneau A, et al. The efficacy of oral splints in the treatment of myofascial pain of the jaw muscles: a controlled clinical trial. Pain 1994;56:85–94.

[48] Ozcelik O, Haytac MC, Seydaoglu G. Immediate post-operative effects of different periodontal treatment modalities on oral health-related quality of life: a randomized clinical trial. J Clin Periodontol 2007;34:788–96.

[49] Walker RJ, Kiyak HA. The impact of providing dental services to frail older adults: perception of elders in adult day health centers. Spec Care Dentist 2007;27:139–43.

[50] Oliver RJ, Clarkson JE, Conway DI, et al. Interventions for the treatment of oral and oropharyngeal cancers: surgical treatment. Cochrane Database Syst Rev 2007;4:CD006205. doi: 10.1002/14651858.CD006205.pub2.

[51] Kujan O, Glenny AM, Oliver RJ, et al. Screening programmes for the early detection and prevention of oral cancer. Cochrane Database Syst Rev 2006;3:CD004150. doi: 10.1002/14651858.CD004150.pub2.

[52] Hita Iglesias C, Prados Atienza MB, Bravo M, et al. Impact of public preventive programmes on oral quality of life of 11 to 12-yr-old school students. Med Oral Patol Oral Cir Bucal 2007;12:E408–11.

[53] Centers for Disease Control and Prevention. Recommendations for using fluoride to prevent and control dental caries in the United States. MMWR Recomm Rep 2001;50(RR14):1–42.

[54] Beltran-Aguilar ED, Griffin S, Lockwood SA. Prevalence and trends in enamel fluorosis in the United States from the 1930s to the 1980s. J Am Dent Assoc 2002;133:157–65.

[55] Rozier RG. The prevalence and severity of enamel fluorosis in North American children. J Public Health Dent 1999;59:239–46.

[56] Public Health Service Committee to Coordinate Environmental Health and Related Programs. Review of fluoride: benefits and risk. Washington, DC: US Department of Health and Human Services, Public Health Service; 1991.

[57] Diefenbach VL, Nevitt GA, Frankel JM. Fluoridation and the appearance of teeth. J Am Dent Assoc 1965;71:1129–37.

[58] Riordan PJ. Perceptions of dental fluorosis. J Dent Res 1993;79:1268–74.

[59] Clark DC, Hann HJ, Williamson MJ, et al. Aesthetic concerns of children and parents in relation to different classifications of the Tooth Surface Index of Fluorosis. Community Dent Oral Epidemiol 1993;21:360–4.

[60] Clark DC. Evaluation of aesthetics for the different classifications of the Tooth Surface Index of Fluorosis. Community Dent Oral Epidemiol 1995;23:80–3.

[61] Ellwood RP, O'Mullane D. Enamel opacities and dental esthetics. J Public Health Dent 1995;60:315–20.

[62] Hawley GM, Ellwood RP, Davies RM. Dental caries, fluorosis and the cosmetic implications of different TF scores in 14-year-old adolescents. Community Dent Health 1996;13:189–92.

[63] Woodward GL, Main PA, Leske JL. Clinical determinants of a parent's satisfaction with the appearance of a child's teeth. Community Dent Oral Epidemiol 1996;24:416–8.

[64] Clark DC, Berkowitz J. The influence of various fluoride exposures on the prevalence of esthetic problems resulting from dental fluorosis. J Public Health Dent 1997;57:144–9.

[65] Lalumandier JA, Rozier RG. Parents' satisfaction with children's tooth color: fluorosis as a contributing factor. J Am Dent Assoc 1998;129:1000–6.

[66] McKnight CB, Levy SM, Cooper SE, et al. A pilot study of esthetic perceptions of dental fluorosis versus selected other dental conditions. ASDC J Dent Child 1998;65:233–8.

[67] Stephen KW, Macpherson LMD, Gilmour WH, et al. A blind caries and fluorosis prevalence study of school-children in naturally fluoridated and nonfluoridated townships of Moray-shire, Scotland. Community Dent Oral Epidemiol 2002;30:70–9.

[68] Levy SM, Warren JJ, Broffitt B, et al. Factors associated with parents' esthetic perceptions of children's mixed dentition fluorosis and demarcated opacities. Pediatr Dent 2005;27:486–92.

[69] Shulman JD, Maupome G, Clark DC, et al. Perceptions of desirable tooth color among parents, dentists and children. J Am Dent Assoc 2004;135:595–604.

[70] Do LG, Spencer AJ. Risk-benefit balance in the use of fluoride among young children. J Dent Res 2007;86:723–8.

[71] Do LG, Spencer AJ. Oral health-related quality of life of children by dental caries and fluorosis experience. J Public Health Dent 2007;67:132–9.

[72] Jokovic A, Locker D, Stephens M, et al. Validity and reliability of a questionnaire for measuring child oral-health related quality of life. J Dent Res 2002;81:459–63.

[73] Jokovic A, Locker D, Tompson B, et al. Questionnaire for measuring global health-related quality of life in eight- to ten-year-old children. Pediatr Dent 2004;26:512–8.

[74] Jokovic A, Locker D, Stephens M, et al. Measuring parental perceptions of child oral health-related quality of life. J Public Health Dent 2003;63:67–72.

[75] Allen PF. Assessment of oral health related quality of life. Health Qual Life Outcomes 2003; 1:40.

[76] Donaldson MS. Using patient-reported outcomes in clinical oncology practice: benefits, challenges and next steps. Expert Review of Pharmacoeconomics and Outcomes Research 2006;6:87–95.

[77] Newsome PR, McGrath C. Patient-centered measures in dental practice: 1. Overview. Dent Update 2006;33:596–8, 600.

[78] Fernandes MJ, Ruta DA, Ogden GR, et al. Assessing oral health-related quality of life in general dental practice in Scotland: validation of OHIP-14. Community Dent Oral Epidemiol 2006;34:53–62.

[79] McGrath C, Newsome PR. Patient-centred measures in dental practice: 2. Quality of life. Dent Update 2007;34:41–2, 44.

[80] Bader JD, Shugars DA, White BA, et al. Development of effectiveness of care and use of services measures for dental care plans. J Public Health Dent 1999;59:142–9.

[81] Leatherman S, McCarthy D. Quality of health care for children and adolescents: a chart-book. New York: The Commonwealth Fund; 2004.

[82] Brown JA, Hays RD, Crall JJ. Summary of cognitive interviews for CAHPS dental care project. Los Angeles (CA): RAND Health; working paper series. WR-101-AHRQ; 2003.

[83] California Healthy Families Program. 2004 report of consumer survey of dental plans. Data Insights Report No. 20, 2004.

[84] Keller S, Evensen CT, Shore K. The TRICARE Dental CAHPS pilot project survey. Final report on year 1 activities. Sliver Spring (MD): American Institutes for Research Health Program; 2005.

ELSEVIER
SAUNDERS

THE DENTAL
CLINICS
OF NORTH AMERICA

Dent Clin N Am 52 (2008) 367–386

Understanding Measurement of Dental Diseases and Research Participation in Practice Set-Up

Amit Chattopadhyay, PhD, MPH, MDS, BDS(Hons)[a,b,*], Oscar Arevalo, DDS, ScD, MBA, MS[c], Woosung Sohn, DDS, MS, PhD, DrPH[d,e]

[a]Department of Epidemiology, University of Kentucky College of Public Health, Room # 209-C, 121 Washington Avenue, Lexington, KY 40536, USA
[b]Division of Dental Public Health, Department of Oral Health Sciences, University of Kentucky College of Dentistry, Lexington, KY, USA
[c]Division of Dental Public Health, College of Dentistry, University of Kentucky, Suite 101, 333 Waller Avenue, Lexington, KY 40504, USA
[d]Department of Cariology, Restorative Sciences and Endodontics, Health Services and Epidemiology Research Unit, Room B305, University of Michigan School of Dentistry, 1011 N. University Avenue, Ann Arbor, MI 48109-1078, USA
[e]Department of Epidemiology, University of Michigan School of Public Health, Ann Arbor, MI, USA

Determination of disease status requires precise judgment. The process of disease determination, referred to as "diagnosis" [1], requires a sound and up-to-date understanding of the nature of the disease that is being measured. As our scientific understanding of the various disease processes increase, clearer definitions, precise diagnostic criteria, appropriate therapeutic rationale, and more effective treatment options are conceived and operationalized. Clinicians make diagnostic judgments and treatment decisions based on the consideration of a predefined set of signs and symptoms, and usually one or more diagnostic tests based on scientific evidence and experience. After diagnoses are made and clear-cut treatment options prescribed, treatment options may need to be modified or selected from several alternative options based on factors not directly related to the disease, such as including socio-demographic characteristics of the patient, societal consensus, and available resources, as well as the severity and prevalence of the disease in the

* Corresponding author. Department of Epidemiology, University of Kentucky College of Public Health, Room # 209-C, 121 Washington Avenue, Lexington, KY 40536.
E-mail address: achat4@email.uky.edu (O. Chattopadhyay).

0011-8532/08/$ - see front matter © 2008 Elsevier Inc. All rights reserved.
doi:10.1016/j.cden.2007.12.005

dental.theclinics.com

community. As much as this decision should be based on scientific evidence, it may also be subjective and vary by individual cases. Measuring a disease level in a population such as in epidemiologic studies, on the other hand, requires a more objective and standardized criteria, so the results can be compared over time, place, and between different populations.

Understanding of oral diseases has increased vastly over the past 150 years. During this period, significant technical advances have been made and substantial changes in disease distribution have been observed [2]. These changes need to be incorporated in measurement of the disease and include new disease definitions, new diagnostic criteria, adoption of new technology, and determination of disease activity [3,4]. This article describes the measurement issues pertaining to three important dental diseases—dental caries, periodontal disease, and dental fluorosis—and expounds the available resources for oral health data and how practicing clinicians can contribute to research using newly developing networks.

Measuring dental caries

Dental caries is the destruction of the dental hard tissue resulting from localized acidic by-products from bacterial fermentation of dietary carbohydrates [5,6]. For a long time, the term dental caries has been used synonymously with frank cavities, despite early precavitated carious lesions on enamel being recognized in the late nineteenth century [2]. Currently, dental caries is understood to involve a continuum of disease states, ranging from initial subclinical, subsurface changes to later stages of clinically detectable lesions manifesting as small cavities that may have significant dentinal involvement at still later stages [7,8].

Caries measurement criteria and clinical implication

In 2004, the International Consensus Workshop on Caries Clinical Trials (ICW-CCT) clarified the meaning of caries diagnosis (which implies a human professional summation of all available data), and further differentiated it to lesion detection (which implies some objective method of determining whether or not disease is present) and lesion assessment (which aims to characterize or monitor a lesion once it has been detected) [9]. From here on, this article will follow the ICW-CCT terminology.

Dental clinicians have been trained to diagnose, detect, and treat "cavities" with the focus of stopping further progression of disease and restoring damaged hard tissue and functionality at the postcavitated phase. Similarly, epidemiologic studies have also measured and reported prevalence of dental caries in population groups using presence of "cavity" as a measurement [10,11]. This basis of clinical dental care, starting in the early and mid twentieth century, was initiated and sustained in industrialized countries that experienced very high levels of prevalence and incidence of dental caries.

This seemed a reasonable approach, considering the ubiquity of severe disease (cavities) and the relatively fast progression of a caries lesion to form a cavity and finally involve the pulp tissue (as is the situation in developing countries, and also in high-risk groups in developed countries today).

With the introduction of preventive measures, mainly water fluoridation, most industrialized countries have experienced substantial declines in caries prevalence and severity [12,13]. With low prevalence and slow progression of caries, it is seen that precavitated caries (reversible condition) lesions are more prevalent than cavitated lesions (irreversible condition) in these countries today [14]. Therefore, it seems appropriate to also develop criteria to identify caries at earlier stages (precavitated), compared with the traditional overt and irreversible lesion only [15]. Current consensus is to detect dental caries at the precavitated stages [9]. The stage at which caries is measured significantly affects epidemiologic assessments of disease prevalence and treatment need in a population, as well as dental clinicians' practice decisions [8,16].

For example, if only cavitated lesions are counted, and prevalence of precavitated lesions is high, then the reported total prevalence (and incidence) of caries would be low and any preventive policy based on such estimates will ignore preventing precavitated lesions from transforming to the cavitated stages. Alternatively, if both precavitated and cavitated lesions are counted, a correct prevalence and incidence estimate will be obtained for "total caries burden," and a policy based on this estimate will presumably address the issue better. However, because preventive measures (primary, secondary, and tertiary) for precavitated and cavitated lesions are substantially different in conceptualization, planning, resource allocation, resource use, and measurement techniques, clear diagnostic criteria distinguishing these two formats of disease should be applied, and total caries burden should also be categorized by precavitated and cavitated lesion category.

An important issue in caries measurement is the lack of coherent and standardized criteria applicable universally. This leads to miscommunications among clinicians, educators, and researchers, and difficulties in interpretability of data from different studies manifesting as apparently conflicting results from studies and reports. A recent review identified 29 different caries assessment criteria-systems being used and found substantial variability in disease processes measured and ambiguity of disease descriptions [17]. One recent development that addresses this issue is a new caries detection system: the International Caries Detection and Assessment System (ICDAS) [18]. The ICDAS classifies the caries process in fives stages, ranging from first visible signs of caries in enamel to extensive cavity with visible dentin, that reflect different steps in the development of dental caries in tooth surfaces and the different levels of care that would be required, ranging from preventive to operative care. The ICDAS aims to provide a flexible yet consistent platform in caries measurement for clinicians and researchers to choose the stage of caries process and other features that fit the needs of their research or practice. This new system has been field tested for validity and reliability [19].

Accuracy of caries measurement

One important source of potential error in measuring precavitated and cavitated lesion is diagnostic (or detection) accuracy. When caries are measured simply as "cavity" versus "no cavity," diagnostic accuracy of visual examination was estimated in a systematic review as having a sensitivity of 63% and specificity of 89% [20]. Use of a sharp explorer did not seem to add substantial accuracy in diagnosis of caries [21], while visual-tactile examination has a sensitivity of 92% [20]. Accuracy of detecting caries at an early stage (eg, precavitated or early or late cavitated) reportedly has a level of sensitivity (66%) similar to that of determining "cavity," but a specificity of only 69% [20].

The level of specificity indicates the level of false positive diagnoses: for example, 95% specificity means 5% false positive. Given same levels of sensitivity and specificity, positive and negative predictive values change depending on the prevalence of disease in a population [22]. As the prevalence of disease declines, a level of false positive diagnoses translates to a lower level of positive predictive value; in other words, a smaller proportion of individuals who are diagnosed as diseased may actually have the disease, which may result in over-treatments and unnecessary anxiety experienced by the patient (Table 1). This has a direct bearing on how caries is defined and measured in epidemiologic studies (as mentioned above), and research data should be interpreted keeping this source of variation in mind.

Caries measurement and decayed-missing-filled index

The presence of dental caries is summarized as the decayed-missing-filled (DMF) index at an individual or at a group of individuals, such as a community, state, and country. The DMF index is, by definition, a count that can range from 0 up to 32 when applied at the tooth level (ie, DMFT) or from 0 up to 128 when applied to the tooth surface level (ie, DMFS). Since its first

Table 1
Illustration of disease prevalence on PPV of a diagnostic test (Sensitivity = 66%, Specificity = 95%)

Prevalence	PPV	NPV
1%	12%	>99%
5%	41%	98%
10%	59%	96%
20%	81%	89%
50%	93%	74%

Abbreviations: PPV, positive predictive value, or the probability that a person who has a positive test result actually has the disease; NPV, negative predictive value, or the probability that a person who has a negative test result actually is healthy (no disease).

introduction in 1938 [23], the DMF index has been used universally as a dental caries summary measure. Details of the DMF index, especially its limitations, are well summarized by Burt and Eklund [24]. As caries measurement moves toward detection of precavitated or early lesions, there arise two important additional issues with the DMF index: (1) it may not be easily usable to determine restorative or preventive treatment need, and (2) DMF indices from different studies may not be comparable unless detection criteria and examination methods (eg, use of an explorer) are clearly described [25].

The DMF index score indicates a total caries experience of an individual and it gives equal weight to decayed, missing because of caries, filled tooth, or tooth surface. Hence, it does not differentiate untreated decay from a well-restored tooth [24]. Also, applying DMF scores to DMFS has raised concerns of overestimation of the number of tooth surfaces missing because of caries. However, using only DF scores underestimates the disease status [26]. Analytical methods to adjust overestimation of disease by the M-component have been proposed [26,27]. Despite the criticism of its limitations, the DMF index will continue to be used until the criteria for dental caries status is defined more clearly. These limitations underscore the need for a more agreed upon description of caries measurement criteria and examination methods [25–27].

Measuring periodontal disease

The term "periodontal disease" has been historically used to describe diseases of gingiva and periodontal ligament. Gingivitis is an inflammation of the gingival tissues where the junctional epithelium, although affected by the disease, remains attached to the tooth at its original level. Periodontitis is also an inflammatory process characterized by clinical attachment loss, alveolar bone loss, and periodontal pockets with or without gingival inflammation [28–30]. Periodontitis may or may not result as a progression of gingivitis, but not all sites affected by gingivitis transition to periodontitis. Periodontal disease is highly prevalent in older adults in the United States, affecting 34% of Americans 30 years or older [31], and remains to be a major cause of tooth loss in adults both in the United States and throughout the world [32–36].

Gingival disease measurement

Introduced in the 1963, the Gingival Index (GI) of Löe and Silness [37] is still used. The GI scores the gingiva on an ordinal scale of 0 to 3 by probing on the mesial, distal, lingual, and buccal surfaces of the teeth. The GI does not take into consideration profound changes in the periodontal tissues and is sensitive enough to capture differences between groups with incipient and severe gingivitis. However, in the mid ranges of gingivitis, its validity is questionable.

Bleeding after probing has become a standard measure of gingivitis in studies, because visual evaluations of inflammation are subjective and conducive to bias. However, the validity of the probing has also been questioned as the pressure applied by different examiners during probing can vary drastically, ranging from 3 g to 130 g depending on the examiner [38]. Gingival probing is not recommended for screenings, surveys, or surveillance because these programs do not require this level of sensitivity, there are concerns about infection control, and bleeding indexes have vague discriminatory power in field studies [39].

Periodontal disease measurement

Initial epidemiologic studies of periodontal diseases used radiographic assessments of alveolar bone loss [40,41]. However, the use of radiographs requires strict standardization of radiographic techniques across clinics and research centers for appropriate comparison of resultant data. Such standardization is difficult to achieve and concerns were raised over ethical issues of exposing participants with radiation. These issues led to the development of more convenient indexes. In the 1960s, the Periodontal Index (PI) introduced by Russell [42] was perceived as an ideal field index and used in epidemiologic studies. The United States Public Health Service agencies measured periodontal disease status in their surveillance activities using the PI until the 1980s. Current understanding of periodontal disease has led to identification of certain deficiencies of the PI. For example, the PI did not include an assessment of clinical attachment loss and graded all pockets of 3 mm or larger equally, combining both gingivitis and periodontitis on the same scale. During the late 1970s there was consensus among many researchers that accurate disease surveillance should include a site-specific measuring as well as clinical attachment loss to represent periodontal disease properly.

The Community Periodontal Index of Treatment Needs (CPITN), introduced by the World Health Organization (WHO) in 1983 [43], included periodontal probing on 10 index teeth. The CPITN has been used as a mechanism to assess treatment needs in most countries throughout the world [44]. Methodologic and theoretic issues have been raised against the CPITN. For example, the CPITN treats gingivitis and periodontitis in the same scale following the paradigm that periodontitis is merely an extension of gingivitis. As a result, the CPITN is not indicated as a tool to assess prevalence of periodontal disease [45–49].

Carlos and colleagues introduced the Extent and Severity Index (ESI) in 1986 [50], attempting to summarize both the extent and the average severity of disease within the group being studied. The ESI uses estimates of attachment level from probing measurements of 14 sites in a quadrant in the maxillary arch and 14 in the contralateral mandibular arch. The ESI is not really an index but a method of summarizing data that permits comparisons among different epidemiologic studies.

A contentious issue that has dogged periodontal disease measurement has been which teeth should be measured for obtaining a true disease burden estimate by maximizing examination efficiency. The ideal solution would be to measure the entire periodontium, checking every available periodontal tissue point. However, it was recognized very early that such an exercise would be very inefficient and consume enormous time and resources, making the examination prohibitively expensive to conduct. Therefore, interest has always been keen to find a way to measure periodontal disease accurately with a resource-conserving paradigm.

In 1951, Ramfjord proposed the Periodontal Disease Index (PDI), which was perhaps a more sensitive version of the PI [51]. Because the PDI is a composite index, it had the same weaknesses as the PI. As a result, the PDI is not longer used. However, Ramfjord's legacy includes the indirect method of measuring clinical attachment loss he described and the partial mouth recording or "Ramfjord teeth," a set of six teeth presumed to the represent the entire mouth during examination (teeth numbers: 3, 9, 12, 19, 25, and 28). Whether the assumption of representation of the dentition for measuring periodontitis is valid or not is being assessed by several studies.

A truer and more exemplative representation of periodontal disease burden in the mouth seems to be obtained through random sampling of measurable sites in the mouth rather than through a fixed set of teeth. A recent study evaluated the bias and precision of probing depth and clinical attachment level estimates of fixed partial examination methods (for example, Ramfjord teeth) and randomly selected sites in the mouth, compared with full-mouth examinations [52]. Among the fixed site methods, Ramfjord's method had the least bias and best representation of periodontal disease in the mouth. However, compared with a method of selecting 36 sites in the mouth randomly, Ramfjord's teeth method had greater bias and relative error. Thus, randomly selected sites provide a better picture of the true burden of periodontal disease in the mouth compared with any fixed site-based measurement method. However, the study noted that both methods underestimated prevalence of periodontal disease; still, random site selection methods were less likely to underestimate prevalence than fixed site based methods. Because of these promising results in favor of random site selection methods, further development of these methods can be expected in the future.

Periodontal disease surveillance

National estimates of periodontal disease prevalence in the United States were calculated for the first time based on the information from the National Health Examination Survey, which included an assessment of periodontal status using the PI [53]. The National Health Examination Survey, which was later renamed as the National Health and Nutrition Examination Survey (NHANES), did not include an oral examination during NHANES II (1976–1980). Instead, the National Center for Health Statistics conducted a periodontal assessment of a subgroup of the Hispanic Population. The

Hispanic Health and Nutrition Examination Survey (1982 and 1984) assessed the periodontal status of the Hispanic population using the PI. At this point the use of the PI to measure periodontal status in national surveys was discontinued. NHANES III (1988–1994) assessed periodontal status by recording probing depths, loss of attachment, and presence of calculus and bleeding in a partial mouth examination.

Surveillance of periodontal status in the United States ceased in the National Health Interview Survey because of the extensive resources required for conducting the clinical examinations. Data collected in NHANES have been used to gain a better understanding of the association between periodontal disease and systemic conditions, including tobacco, heart attack, and cardiovascular disease. Despite the clinical value of the data generated, the surveillance as conducted had limitations. The use of partial mouth evaluations might have led to misrepresentation of the true prevalence of periodontal disease [54,55]. Partial versus full-mouth assessment and fixed site versus randomly selected sites for periodontal disease assessment have been discussed above. The clinical examination process for conducting periodontal assessment in NHANES and other surveys was a very resource-intensive process. In 2005 with a funding reduction in place, the clinical periodontal assessment was eliminated in NHANES [53]. As a result, surveillance for periodontal diseases is almost nonexistent at state, county, or local levels in the United States [56].

A potential alternative to overcome these problems is the use of self-reported periodontal disease status assessment in population surveys. In 2003, the Centers for Disease Control and Prevention (CDC), in conjunction with the American Academy of Periodontology convened a conference, where the importance of periodontal disease surveillance and its potential association with systemic diseases were discussed. A panel of experts was formed to make recommendations for alternative mechanisms to assess periodontal disease that could be integrated into existing surveillance. In particular, the panel was to determine whether self-reported measures could be valid to predict the prevalence of periodontal disease and to develop and test questions to be used to survey the United States population [57].

The inexpensiveness and convenience of self-reports measures are appealing for health surveillance and forecasting health outcomes. For example, since 1984 the CDC has used self-reported questions to track chronic diseases and risk behaviors among the United States populations as part of the Behavioral Risk Factor Surveillance System, with compelling evidence for high reliability and validity [58]. However, using self-reported measures to estimate the prevalence of periodontal disease presents several challenges [48]. For example, because periodontal disease is in many cases an asymptomatic process, individuals affected by periodontal disease may be unaware of the condition [59]. Therefore, disease prevalence may be underestimated because asymptomatic individuals are unaware of their disease status. Individuals learn about their disease once they are informed by their dentist [60,61].

However, the resource conservative nature is a strong argument in favor of using periodontal disease status self-report as a method to estimate periodontal disease prevalence for surveillance purpose, and is currently being field tested by the CDC. The initial step of the CDC Periodontal Disease Surveillance Project consisted of a thorough review of the literature of previous studies that measured the validity of self-reported measures to predict the prevalence of periodontal disease [62]. Based on the results of this review, the workgroup focused on exploring the use of combined self-reported measures (gum disease, bone loss, history of treatment of gum disease, history of loose teeth, use of mouth wash or dental rinse, and cleaning between teeth) and known risk factors (age, smoking, and diabetes) to predict the prevalence of periodontitis among the population [63]. As a set of promising self-reported questions that showed evidence of being valid predictors of periodontal disease prevalence within populations were derived from a range of existing datasets analyzed by the panel experts. The validity of six periodontal screening questions were assessed as part of the Australian National Survey of Adult Oral Health, a population based survey in Australia that has interview and clinical protocols similar to NHANES.

The Australian study concluded that the questions could be used in large population surveys, attaining useful levels of validity in predicting the prevalence of clinically evaluated periodontal disease [64]. After testing for comprehension in the United States the workgroup made slight modifications to the language and format and a set eight questions were adopted for further testing in a pilot study (Box 1) [65]. The National Center for Health Statistics is conducting the study using NHANES protocols for interviews and clinical examinations, including a full-mouth examination. If the pilot study proves to be successful, the valid questions will be incorporated into NHANES 2009–2010 [63].

Measuring dental fluorosis

Dental fluorosis is defined as a hypomineralization of the enamel produced by excessive ingestion of fluoride during development stages of the tooth [66]. The enamel surface and subsurface present increase porosity, resulting in a clinical appearance that varies from barely noticeable white flecks to severe brown staining. A longitudinal study conducted by the National Institutes of Dental and Craniofacial Research (NIDCR) found that the prevalence of fluorosis in seven areas where the water supply was optimally fluoridated did not increase over a 10-year period (1980–1990), suggesting that the increase was caused by the availability of fluoride in sources other than drinking water [67]. Several indexes that describe the clinical appearance of dental fluorosis have been developed over the past several decades. This article includes only those indices that have been widely used.

In the original form of the Fluorosis Index (FI), Dean [68] categorized fluorosis on a seven-point ordinal scale that ranged from normal to severe,

Box 1. Self-report questions to the prevalence of periodontal disease in the United States population to be used in the 2009–2010 NHANES*

Gum disease is a common problem with the mouth. People with gum disease might have swollen gums, receding gums, sore or infected gums, or loose teeth.

PB1: Do you think you might have gum disease?
1 = Yes
2 = No
7 = Refused
9 = Don't Know

PB2: Overall, how would you rate the health of your teeth and gums?
1 = Excellent
2 = Very good
3 = Good
4 = Fair
5 = Poor
7 = Refused
9 = Don't Know

PB3: Have you ever had treatment for gum disease, such as scaling and root planning, sometimes called "deep cleaning"?
1 = Yes
2 = No
7 = Refused
9 = Don't Know

PB4: Have you ever had any teeth become loose on their own, without an injury?
1 = Yes
2 = No
7 = Refused
9 = Don't Know

PB5: Have you ever been told by a dental professional that you lost bone around your teeth?
1 = Yes
2 = No
7 = Refused
9 = Don't Know

(*continued on next page*)

PB6: During the past 3 months, have you noticed a tooth that doesn't look right?
1 = Yes
2 = No
7 = Refused
9 = Don't Know

PB7: Aside from brushing your teeth with a toothbrush, in the last 7 days, how many times did you use dental floss or any other device to clean between your teeth?
___: Number of days
77 = Refused

PB8: Aside from brushing your teeth with a toothbrush, in the last 7 days, how many times did you use mouthwash or other dental rinse product that you use to treat dental disease or dental problems?
___: Number of days
77 = Refused

---

* Personal Communication, Dr Bruce Dye. Centers for Disease Control and Prevention, National Center for Health Statistics.

---

based on clinical examinations conducted on approximately 2,000 individuals. Thereafter, Dean revised the FI after assessing more than 10,000 individuals. Specifically, he merged the "moderately severe" and "severe" categories into a single "severe" category, resulting in the six-category measurement currently used [69]. Dean's FI has been criticized because it does not provide information about the distribution of fluorosis within the dentition. Furthermore, the "questionable" category is considered diagnostically ambiguous and the index lacks sensitivity in the higher categories. However, Dean's FI has been widely used in epidemiologic studies around the world, and therefore, is of value when making comparisons.

The Tooth Surface Index of Fluorosis (TSIF) was introduced by researchers of the NIDCR in 1984 when they assessed the prevalence of dental caries and dental fluorosis in communities that had optimal and above-optimal concentrations of natural fluoride in drinking water [70,71]. The TSIF assigns a score ranging from 0 to 7 to the facial and lingual surfaces of anterior teeth and to the buccal, occlusal, and lingual surface of posterior teeth. The TSIF seems to have two advantages over Dean's index: the first is its unambiguous scoring system and the second is its scoring of surfaces rather than individual teeth [72]. The TSIF seems to be more sensitive than Dean's index in identifying the mildest forms of fluorosis. However, the WHO still recommends use of Dean's Index in its basic survey manual [73].

Dean's Index has been modified to meet specific needs. For example, the Thylstrup-Fejerskov Index (TFI) was developed based on the need to measure enamel changes in areas where fluoride in drinking water was at higher levels than those studied by Dean [74]. TFI includes a 10-point ordinal scale classifying enamel changes related to increased fluoride exposure. As originally developed, occlusal and facial surfaces were scored in the TFI; however, as the scores on the two surfaces tend to be similar, most investigators use only one surface.

The Fluorosis Risk Index (FRI) was introduced in 1990 [75]. The objective of the FRI is to improve the ability to relate the risk of fluorosis to the developmental stage of the permanent dentition at the time of exposure to fluoride. The FRI is distinctive in that each tooth is assessed for fluorosis on four enamel zones, and it selectively classifies each zone into one of two zones: FRI-I and FRI-II zones. FRI-I includes 10 early developing zones (occlusal cusp areas of first molars and incisal edges of 6 of the 8 incisors). FRI-II includes 24 zones, which develop and erupt later. The FRI has great potential for use in analytic epidemiologic studies to permit an accurate identification of association between age and ingestion of fluoride and the development of fluorosis on permanent teeth [76].

The difficulty in differentiating between fluoride and nonfluoride defects and the confusion in the classifications of mottled enamel, dental fluorosis, and other enamel defects led to the development of a second group of indices covering all types of defects [77–80]. The development of these numerous indices led to the creation of the Developmental Defects of Dental Enamel (DDE) index, with the objective to avoid confusion in reporting results of enamel defects and fluorosis [81]. The DDE has been used in studies in Europe and New Zealand [82,83]; however, the large amount of data generated has resulted in difficulty presenting results in a consequential manner.

Monitoring of oral health status of a population

Disease measurement and public health

The core functions of public health include assessment, policy development, and assurance [84]. The assessment—regular collection and dissemination of data of health status, community health needs, and epidemiologic issues—enables the latter steps and therefore provides fundamental basis for successful public health practice. These profound goals of assessment aim to understand the disease distribution in populations and to explain the causes or determinants of the disease, so that planning for and implementation of policy or program to control and prevent the disease is achievable.

The CDC maintains a comprehensive searchable Web site of Mortality and Morbidity Weekly Reports, and its special series reports (SS-), which includes several reports related to oral health [85]. Several other important reports can be downloaded from Web sites of related professional organizations. For example, the Future of Dentistry Report can be downloaded from the American Dental Association's Web site [86], and the Surgeon General's Report on Oral Health is available at the Department of Health and Human Services Web page [87]. Whereas these reports are freely available, one of the key problem elements in dental public health research is to obtain, assess, and analyze oral health data of populations, to make inferences about and develop suitable strategies to improve oral health of the populations.

Oral health data sources

Several national surveys are conducted that include some basic oral health related information, such as the Behavioral Risk Factor Surveillance System, NHANES (currently the fourth survey is ongoing), National Health Interview Survey, Medical Expenditure Panel Survey, Surveillance, Epidemiology, and End Results, and a series of surveys conducted by the NIDCR. Data for these surveys are public-use data and available from their respective Web sites. The NIDCR also maintains a directory of usable dental data that can be obtained on CD-ROM from their office. However, there is a shortage of local-level data (ie, state-level, and especially county level data). Several states run their surveillance programs periodically to collect oral health related data. These states feed the data to a central point to disseminate basic information about the status of oral health in the state, which forms the National Oral Health Surveillance System (NOHSS).

National Oral Health Surveillance System

The NOHSS was established in 2001 and is a collaborative effort between the CDC's Division of Oral Health and the Association of State and Territorial Dental Directors. NOHSS is designed to monitor the burden of oral disease, use of the oral health care delivery system, and the status of community water fluoridation on both a national and state level [88]. NOHSS includes indicators of oral health, information on state dental programs, and links to other important sources of oral health information.

Oral health indicators in NOHSS

A total of eight oral health indicators that NOHSS covers include: dental visit, teeth cleaning, complete tooth loss, loss of six or more teeth, fluoridation status, dental sealants, caries experience, untreated tooth decay, and cancer of the oral cavity and pharynx. The NOHSS Web site allows interactively querying the database for national and state level information by years (where data is available), and also informs the user from which survey the statistic was calculated. It also includes basic Web-based national and state-level maps for the indicators recorded, apart from including synopses of state and territorial dental public health programs [88]. Therefore, one can compare state estimates with national or those of other states for one of the indicators covered.

Data tables for oral health indicators

The NIDCR and CDC Dental, Oral, and Craniofacial Data Resource Center maintains the Catalog of Surveys and Archive of Procedures Related to Oral Health [89] that provides selected data tables from different years (national and state). Recent updates are provided for each of the oral health indicators in both HTML and PDF formats that can be viewed, saved, and printed from the Web site [89]. This catalog includes examined indicators, such as dental caries, oral and pharyngeal cancers, periodontal assessment and disease, sealants, smokeless tobacco lesions, tooth loss, and self-reported indicators such as dental visits, self-assessed oral health status, usual source of dental care, orofacial pain, tobacco use, and dental insurance.

Role of dental practitioners outside academia in dental research

In March of 2005, the NIDCR announced it had awarded three grants, totaling $75 million, that establish regional "practice-based" research networks (PBRN) to investigate with greater scientific rigor "everyday" issues in the delivery of oral health care [90]. The goal of PBRNs is to encourage practicing dentists and hygienists to propose and conduct each clinical study in close collaboration with their network colleagues. The general idea of developing the PBRNs is to address practical, real-world issues, and generate data that will be of immediate interest to practitioners and their patients [90]. Recently, a group of dental practitioners participating in the PBRN effort wrote about their perspective, calling the effort to be a "win-win for private-practice dentists and the future of dentistry" [91]. Although not enough data is available at this moment about success or utility of PBRNs in dentistry, such networks have been in existence in medical research for over two decades; they have generally been successful and have resulted in significant clinical protocol changes [92].

All treatments carry risks, and these risks may vary depending upon practices because of practitioner experience variability or even because of patients' biologic response or compliance with treatment and oral hygiene maintenance variability. The real-world situation in which the private practitioner works may vary substantially from the clinical or device trial environment where the drugs and devices are comprehensively tested. Therefore, the practitioner needs to develop a guideline for accepting those treatment protocols that would work in their practice situation. Such practice of evidence-based dentistry shifts the responsibility of selecting practice-appropriate treatments to the practitioner. The selection may be done after assessing the risks and benefits for the patient pool that the practitioner manages, but only after developing enough evidence for adopting these strategies or protocols.

Two broad types of approaches may be adopted for incorporating new techniques in practice: a precautionary approach and a risk-based approach. The precautionary approach would seek evidence for each available alternative and use the one with minimum risk, whereas the alternative approach would use any alternative until adverse events occur [93]. Therefore, the "precautionary principle" calls for preventive actions in the face of uncertain information about risks [94]. The precautionary principle is put to use when there is a basis for hypothesizing an impact on health from a given exposure, but available epidemiologic data do not clearly support or refute such a hypothesis [95]. Applying precaution requires thinking more broadly about risks, taking an interdisciplinary approach to science and policy, and considering a wide range of alternatives to potentially harmful activities. The precautionary principle is not at odds with, but rather complements evidence-based practice in situations of scientific uncertainty and complex risks [94].

With emphasis on PBRNs, there is a need for private practitioners to incorporate evidence-based practice principles in their daily work schedules. Private practitioners may also become actively involved with reporting adverse events and in reporting device malfunction or design to the Food and Drug Administration [96] to help improve device design and effectiveness. At the same time, these practitioners participating in PBRNs will also need to update their understanding of research methods and scientific inference-making to be able to contribute substantially to the improvement of oral health care delivery.

One opinion suggests that the key problems in involving the private practitioner in PBRNs is having enough time to do a good job for the patients and to manage the clinical research projects at the same time [97]. To make this happen, it has been suggested that the practice staff must be educated and they must buy into the concept. For this to happen, they must be given time to acclimatize to the requirements of practice based research.

How should the private practitioner integrate the PBRN? Apart from getting some training in research methods, the first thing that a practitioner should do is to enlist the help of experienced research investigators [97,98]. With the proper background, experience, support staff, and commitment, private dental practitioners can contribute significantly to research and science [98].

Summary

A general understanding of the measurement of dental diseases can help practitioners and their patients in different ways. Knowledge of the patient's past and current disease status, compared with others of the same gender and age, is a valuable first step in the process of assessing the patient's future risk of disease. Understanding of oral diseases, their etiologic factors, and treatment methods, has increased vastly during the last century. Similarly, measuring criteria for epidemiologic purposes has evolved based on new knowledge, particular clinical questions, and applicability in field studies. The availability of multiple criteria systems has led to an inability to compare results from different studies. Therefore, an important issue in oral health disease management is the lack of standardized criteria applicable universally. Clinical measurement of oral health diseases as part of survey and surveillance is a costly endeavor because of the extensive resources required. In the future, epidemiologic studies might rely more heavily on less expensive approaches, such as self-reported questions. Practicing dentists might play a more significant role in research as clinical studies shift from the traditional academic setting to practice-based networks. To critically interpret data as it becomes available, these practitioners will need to update their understanding of epidemiologic principles and research methods.

References

[1] Last JM. A dictionary of epidemiology. 4th edition. New York: Oxford University Press; 2001.
[2] Ismail AI, Hasson H, Sohn W. Dental caries in the second millennium. J Dent Educ 2001; 65(10):953–9.
[3] Whelton H. Overview of the impact of changing global patterns of dental caries experience on caries clinical trials. J Dent Res 2004;83(Spec Iss C):C29–34.
[4] ten Bosch JJ, Angmar-Mansson B. Characterization and validation of diagnostic methods. Monogr Oral Sci 2000;17:174–89.
[5] Fejerskov O, Kidd EAM. Dental caries: the disease and its clinical management. Copenhagen, Denmark: Munksgaard; 2003.
[6] Thylstrup A. When is caries caries, and what should we do about it? Quintessence Int 1998; 29:594–8.
[7] Kidd EAM, Fejerskov O. What constitutes dental caries? Histopathology of carious enamel and dentin related to the action of cariogenic biofilms. J Den Res 2004;83:C35–8.
[8] Pitts NB. Modern concepts of caries measurement. J Dent Res 2004;83(Spec No C):C43–7.
[9] Pitts NB, Stamm JW. International consensus workshop on caries clinical trials (ICW-CCT)—final consensus statements: agreeing where the evidence leads. J Dent Res 2004; 83(Spec No C):C125–8.
[10] World Health Organization, Oral health surveys. Basic methods. 4th edition. Geneva: World Health Organization; 1997.
[11] National Institute for Dental and Craniofacial Research (NIDCR). Oral Health of United States Adults. Bethesda (MD): NIDCR; 1987. p. 161–5.
[12] Marthaler TM. Changes in dental caries 1953–2003. Caries Res 2004;38:173–81.
[13] Petersen PE. The World Oral Health Report 2003: continuous improvement of oral health in the 21st century—the approach of the WHO Global Oral Health Programme. Community Dent Oral Epidemiol 2003;31(Suppl 1):3–23.
[14] Ismail AI. Clinical diagnosis of precavitated carious lesions. Community Dent Oral Epidemiol 1997;25(1):13–23.
[15] Bader JD, Brown JP. Dilemmas in caries diagnosis. J Am Dent Assoc 1993;124:48–50.
[16] Rimmer PA, Pitts NB. Effects of diagnostic threshold and overlapped approximal surfaces on reported caries status. Community Dent Oral Epidemiol 1991;16:166–70.
[17] Ismail A. Visual and visuo-tactile detection of dental caries. J Den Res 2004;83(Spec Iss C): C56–66.
[18] Pitts NB. "ICDAS"—an international system for caries detection and assessment being developed to facilitate caries epidemiology, research and appropriate clinical management. Community Dent Health 2004;21:193–8.

[19] Ismail AI, Sohn W, Tellez M, et al. The international caries detection and assessment system (ICDAS): an integrated system for measuring dental caries. Community Dent Oral Epidemiol 2007;35(3):170–8.

[20] Bader JD, Shugars DA, Bonito AJ. Systematic reviews of selected dental caries diagnostic and management methods. J Dent Educ 2001;65(10):960–8.

[21] Lussi A. Validity of diagnostic and treatment decisions of fissure caries. Caries Res 1991;25: 296–303.

[22] Fletcher RW, Fletcher SW. Clinical epidemiology: The essentials. 4th edition. Baltimore: Lippincott Williams & Wilkins; 2005.

[23] Klein H, Palmer CE, Knutson JW. Studies on dental caries: I. dental status and dental needs of elementary school children. Public Health Rep 1938;53:751–65.

[24] Burt BA, Eklund SE. Dentistry, Dental Practice, and the Community. 6th edition. Philadelphia: Elsevier Saunders; 2005.

[25] Burt BA. How useful are cross-sectional data from surveys of dental caries? Community Dent Oral Epidemiol 1997;25:36–41.

[26] Lawrence HP, Beck JD, Hunt RJ, et al. Adjustment of the M-component of the DMFS index for prevalence studies of older adults. Community Dent Oral Epidemiol 1996;24:322–31.

[27] Boradbent JM, Thomson WM. For debate: problems with the DMF index pertinent to dental caries analysis. Community Dent Oral Epidemiol 2005;33:400–9.

[28] Page RC, Schroeder HE. Pathogenesis of inflammatory periodontal disease. A summary of current work. Lab Invest 1976;33:235–49.

[29] Lindhe J, Okamoto H, Yoneyama T, et al. Longitudinal changes in periodontal disease in untreated subjects. J Clin Periodontol 1989;16:662–70.

[30] Machtei EE, Hausman E, Dunford R, et al. Longitudinal study of predictive factors for periodontal disease and tooth loss. J Clin Periodontol 1999;26:374–80.

[31] Albandar JM, Brunelle JA, Kigngman A. Destructive periodontal disease in adults 30 years of age and older in the United States, 1988–1994. J Periodontol 1999;70:13–29.

[32] Oliver RC, Brown LJ, Löe H. Periodontal diseases in the United States population. J Periodontol 1998;69(2):269–78.

[33] Sheiham A, Netuveli G. Periodontal diseases in Europe. Periodontology 2000;29(1):104–21, 2002.

[34] Corbet EF, Zee KY, Lo EC. Periodontal diseases in Asia and Oceania. Periodontology 2000; 29(1):122–52, 2002.

[35] Ong G. Periodontal disease and tooth loss. Int Dent J 1998;48:233–8.

[36] Irfan UM, Dawson DV, Bissada NF. Epidemiology of periodontal disease: a review and clinical perspectives. J Int Acad Periodontol 2001;3(1):14–21, Review.

[37] Löe H, Silness J. Periodontal disease in pregnancy. I. Prevalence and severity. Acta Odontol Scand 1963;21:533–51.

[38] Polson AM, Caton JG. Current status of bleeding in the diagnosis of periodontal diseases. J Periodontol 1985;56(Spec Issue):1–3.

[39] Macaulay WR, Taylor GO, Lennon MA, et al. The suitability of three periodontal indices for epidemiological studies conducted for planning purposes. Community Dent Health 1998;13:249–57.

[40] Sandler HC, Stahl SS. Measurement of periodontal disease prevalence. J Am Dent Assoc 1959;58:93–7.

[41] Schei O, Waerhaug J, Lovdal A, et al. Alveolar bone loss as related to oral hygiene and age. J Peridontol 1959;30:7–16.

[42] Russell AL. A system of classification and scoring for prevalence surveys of periodontal disease. J Dent Res 1956;35:350–9.

[43] Ainamo J, Barmes D, Beagrie G, et al. Development of the World Health Organization (WHO) Community Periodontal Index of Treatment Needs (CPITN). Int Dent J 1982;32:281–91.

[44] Page RC, Morrison EC. Summary of outcomes and recommendations of the workshop on (CPITN). Int Dent J 1994;44(5 Suppl 1):589–94.

[45] Lewis JM, Morgan MV, Wright FAC. The validity of the CPITN scoring and presentation method for measuring periodontal conditions. J Clin Periodontol 1994;21:1–6.

[46] Rams TE, Listgarten MA, Slots J. Efficacy of CPITN sextant scores for detection of periodontitis disease activity. J Clin Periodontol 1996;23:355–61.

[47] Baelum V, Manji F, Wanzala P, et al. Relationship between CPITN and periodontal attachment loss findings in an adult population. J Clin Periodontol 1995;22:146–52.

[48] Benigeri M, Brodeur J-M, Payette M, et al. Community periodontal index of treatment needs and prevalence of periodontal conditions. J Clin Periodontol 2000;27:308–12.

[49] Kingman A, Albandar JM. Methodological aspects of epidemiological studies of periodontal diseases. Periodontol 2000 2002;29:11 30.

[50] Carlos JP, Wolfe MD, Kingman A. The extent and severity index: a simple method for use in epidemiologic studies of periodontal disease. J Clin Periodontol 1986;13(5):500–5.

[51] Ramfjord SP. Indices for prevalence and incidence of periodontal disease. J Periodontol 1959;30:51–9.

[52] Beck JD, Caplan DJ, Preisser JS, et al. Reducing the bias of probing depth and attachment level estimates using random partial-mouth recording. Community Dent Oral Epidemiol 2006;34:1–10.

[53] Dye BA, Thornton-Evans G. A brief history of national surveillance efforts for periodontal disease in the United States. J Periodontol 2007;78:1373–9.

[54] Slade GD, Beck JD. Plausibility of periodontal disease estimates from NHANES III. J Public Health Dent 1999;59:67–72.

[55] Tomar SL. Public health perspectives on surveillance for periodontal diseases. J Periodontol 2007;78:1380–6.

[56] Page RC, Eke PI. Case definitions for use in population-based surveillance of periodontitis. J Periodontol 2007;78:1387–99.

[57] Eke PI. Public health implications of periodontal infections in adults. Conference proceedings. J Public Health Dent 2005;65:56–65.

[58] National Center for Chronic Disease Prevention and Health Promotion. Behavioral Risk Factor Surveillance System (BRFSS). Available at: http://www.cdc.gov/brfss/. Accessed February 2, 2008.

[59] Pihlstrom BL, Michalowics BS, Johnson NW. Periodontal diseases. Lancet 2005;366: 1809–20.

[60] Drilea SK, Reid BC, Li CH, et al. Dental visits among smoking and nonsmoking US adults in 2000. Am J Health Behav 2005;29:462–71.

[61] Tomar SL, Lester A. Dental and other health care visits among U.S. adults with diabetes. Diabetes Care 2000;23:1505–10.

[62] Blicher B, Joshipura K, Eke PI. Validation of self-reported periodontal disease: A systematic review. J Dent Res 2005;884:881–90.

[63] Eke PI, Genco RJ, Eke PI. CDC periodontal disease surveillance project: background, objectives and progress report. J Periodontol 2007;78:1366–71.

[64] Slade GD. Interim analysis of validity of periodontitis screening questions in the Australian population. J Periodontol 2007;78:1463–70.

[65] Miller K, Eke PI, Schoua-Glusberg A. Cognitive evaluation of self-report questions for surveillance of periodontitis. J Periodontol 2007;78(Suppl 7):1455–62.

[66] Fejerskow O, Manji F, Baelum V. The nature and mechanisms of dental fluorosis in man. J Dent Res 1990;69(Spec Issue):692–700.

[67] Selwitz RH, Nowkjack-Raymer RE, Kingman A, et al. Prevalence of dental caries and dental fluorosis in areas with optimal and above-optimal water fluoride concentrations: a 10-year follow-up survey. J Public Health Dent 1995;55:85–93.

[68] Dean HT. Classification of mottled enamel diagnosis. J Am Dent Assoc 1934;21:1421–6.

[69] Dean HT. The investigation of physiological effects by the epidemiological method. In: Moulton FR, editor. Fluorine and dental health. Washington DC: American Association for the Advancement of Science; 1946. p. 5–31.

[70] Horowitz HS, Driscoll WS, Meyers RJ, et al. A new method for assessing the prevalence of dental fluorosis—the tooth surface index of fluorosis. J Am Dent Assoc 1984;109: 37–41.

[71] Driscoll WS, Horowitz HS, Meyers RJ, et al. Prevalence of dental caries and dental fluorosis in areas with negligible, optimal, and above-optimal fluoride concentrations in drinking water. J Am Dent Assoc 1986;113:29–33.

[72] Rozier RG. Epidemiological indices for measuring the clinical manifestations of dental fluorosis: overview and critique. Adv Dent Res 1994;8(1):39–55.

[73] World Health Organization. Oral health surveys; basic methods. 4th edition. Geneva: WHO; 1997.

[74] Thylstrup A, Fejerskov O. Clinical appearance of dental fluorosis in permanent teeth in relation to histologic changes. Community Dent Oral Epidemiol 1978;6:315–28.

[75] Pendrys DG. The fluorosis risk index: a method for investigating risk factors. J Public Health Dent 1990;50(5):291–9.

[76] Levy SM, Hong L, Warren JJ, et al. Use of the fluorosis risk index in a cohort study: the Iowa fluoride study. J Public Health Dent 2006;66(2):92–6.

[77] Young MA. An epidemiological study of enamel opacities. PhD Thesis. London (UK): University of London; 1973.

[78] Al-Alousi W, Jackson D, Crompton G, et al. Enamel mottling in a fluoride and non-fluoride community, parts. An epidemiological study of enamel opacities. PhD Thesis. London (UK): University of London; 1973.

[79] Jackson D, James PMC, Wolfe WB. Fluoridation in Anglesey, a Clinical Study. Br Dent J 1975;138:165–71.

[80] Murray JJ, Shaw L. Classification and prevalence of enamel opacities in the human deciduous and permanent dentitions. Arch Oral Biol 1979;24:7–12.

[81] Fédération Dentaire Internationale. Commission on oral research and epidemiology. An epidemiological index of developmental defects of dental enamel (DDE index). Int Dent J 1982;32:159–67.

[82] Dummer PM, Kingdon A, Kingdon R. Prevalence of enamel developmental defects in a group of 11- and 12-year-old children in South Wales. Community Dent Oral Epidemiol 1986;14:119–22.

[83] Suckling GW, Pearce IEF. Developmental defects of enamel in a group of New Zealand children. Community Dent Oral Epidemiol 1978;6:315–28.

[84] Institute of Medicine. The future of public health. Washington, DC: National Academy Press; 1988.

[85] CDC. MMWR. Available at: http://www.cdc.gov/mmwr/. Accessed February 2, 2008.

[86] ADA. Future of dentistry. Available at: http://www.ada.org/prof/resources/topics/future dent/index.asp. Accessed February 2, 2008.

[87] Oral Health America. Available at: http://www.surgeongeneral.gov/library/oralhealth/.

[88] CDC. National Oral health surveillance system. Available at: http://www.cdc.gov/nohss/. http://drc.hhs.gov/report/8_1.htm. Accessed February 26, 2007.

[89] NIDCR. The catalog of surveys and archive of procedures related to oral health. NIDCR/ CDC dental, oral and craniofacial data resource center. Available at: http://drc.hhs.gov/ catalog.htm. Accessed February 2, 2008.

[90] NIDCR. NIDCR Awards Grants for New Practice-Based Initiative. Available at: http:// www.nidcr.nih.gov/NewsAndReports/NewsReleases/NewsRelease03312005.htm. Accessed February 2, 2008.

[91] Veitz-Keenan A, Berkowitz GS, Brandes I, et al. Practice-based research networks. NY State Dent J 2007;73(3):14–5.

[92] Moskowitz E. Clinical research in dentistry. NY State Dent J 2007;73(3):4.

[93] Hujoel P. The precautionary principle in dentistry. J Evid Base Dent Pract 2006;6:5.

[94] Tickner J, Coffin M. What does the precautionary principle mean for evidence-based dentistry? J Evid Based Dent Pract 2006;6(1):6–15.

[95] Weiss NS. When can the result of epidemiologic research not eliminate the need to invoke the precautionary principle? J Evid Based Dent Pract 2006;6(1):16–8.

[96] Runner S. FDA marketing claims, and the practitioner. J Evid Based Dent Pract 2006;6(1): 19–23.

[97] Wagenberg BD. Practice-based research: is it worthwhile? A clinician's view. J Evid Based Dent Pract 2006;6(2):164–6.

[98] Lader EW, Cannon CP, Ohman EM, et al. American college of cardiology foundation. The clinician as investigator: participating in clinical trials in the practice setting. Circulation 2004;109(21):2672–9.

ELSEVIER
SAUNDERS

THE DENTAL
CLINICS
OF NORTH AMERICA

Dent Clin N Am 52 (2008) 387–401

Fluorides in Dental Public Health Programs

Jayanth V. Kumar, DDS, MPH[a,b,*],
Mark E. Moss, DDS, MS, PhD[c,d]

[a]Oral Health Surveillance and Research, Bureau of Dental Health, Room 542, ESP Tower,
New York State Department of Health, Albany, NY 12237, USA
[b]School of Public Health, University at Albany, One University
Place Rensselaer, Albany, NY 12144, USA
[c]Bureau of Dental Health, Room 542, ESP Tower, New York State
Department of Health, Albany, NY 12237, USA
[d]InterLakes Health, 1019 Wicker Street, Ticonderoga, NY 12883, USA

Fluorides in dental public health programs

Dental caries is a chronic disease that affects a large proportion of the population in the United States. Although dental caries has declined in the United States, almost 28% of 2- to 5-year-old children experience the disease [1]. Among 16- to 19-year-old children, the average number of decayed, missing, and filled surfaces (DMFS) is 5.8. Adults 40 to 59 years of age have an average of 42 DMFS. Dental diseases account for 30% of all health care expenditures in children [2].

Theoretically, dental caries can be controlled by altering the bacterial flora in the mouth, modifying the diet, increasing the resistance of tooth to acid attack, or reversing the demineralization process. In practice, however, only the use of fluorides and sealants has been shown to be successful in reducing dental caries in populations [2]. Therefore, the development of interventions that employ fluorides to prevent dental caries has been a large part of the dental public health effort. Traditionally, dental public health has focused on the community as a whole instead of the individual patient, and targeted interventions and policies to improve the health of the community. This article reviews some of the ways fluorides are used in public health programs and discusses issues related to the effectiveness, cost, and policy of these uses.

* Corresponding author. Oral Health Surveillance and Research, Bureau of Dental Health, Room 542, ESP Tower, New York State Department of Health, Albany, NY 12237.
E-mail address: jvk01@health.state.ny.us (J.V. Kumar).

0011-8532/08/$ - see front matter. Published by Elsevier Inc.
doi:10.1016/j.cden.2007.11.003

dental.theclinics.com

Fluoride and dental health

Frederick McKay, a Colorado dentist, noticed that clusters of individuals had stained teeth, and he hypothesized that these stains were related to some agent in the drinking water [3]. Studies later identified the agent as the fluoride in water. During the epidemiologic investigations of the staining, H. T. Dean made the observation that children with mottled teeth seemed to have less tooth decay than those who did not have the mottling. Further studies clearly demonstrated the inverse association between the fluoride level in drinking water and the amount of tooth decay [4].

Four large-scale community studies were initiated in the period of 1945 to 1947 to assess whether adjusting the level of fluoride in drinking water to an optimal level could provide a beneficial caries-inhibiting effect. Water supplies in the communities of Grand Rapids, Michigan, Newburgh, New York, Evanston, Illinois, and Brantford, Ontario were adjusted, and this became the birth of fluoridation. The results obtained in these studies were compelling both because of the magnitude of the beneficial impact of fluoride on dental caries and because of the consistency observed across the studies [5]. Since the early studies of water fluoridation, different approaches have been investigated to deliver fluoride to the oral environment, as water fluoridation is not practical in every community. Table 1 shows fluoride levels and the frequency of its use in public health programs.

Mechanism of action of fluoride

The initial studies suggested that the beneficial effects of fluoride were a result of incorporation of fluoride into tooth crystals during its formation [6]. The early studies also showed that there were posteruptive benefits from

Table 1
Use of fluorides in public health programs

Program	Fluoride (F) levels	Frequency
Community water fluoridation	0.7 mg/L –1.2 mg/L F	Daily
School-based fluoride rinse	10 mL or 5 mL 0.2% sodium fluoride (9 mg F per 10 mL)	Weekly
Fluoride tablet	0.25 mg to 1 mg F	Daily
Fluoride varnish	0.3 mL–0.5 mL 5% sodium fluoride per application 22,600 ppm (2.26% F)	3 to 6 month interval
Supervised tooth brushing	1,000 ppm–1,100 ppm (1 mg to 1.1 mg F/g)	Twice daily
Salt fluoridation	200 mg–250 mg F/kg salt	Daily

Data from US Department of Health and Human Services. Oral health in America: A Report of the Surgeon General. Rockville, MD, National Institute of Health; 2000.

fluoridation [4–7]. This led to studies of topical effects of fluoride on the tooth surface. The laboratory studies suggest that the predominant action of fluoride is in the process of remineralization and inhibition of demineralization of enamel [8,9]. However, epidemiologic studies conducted in the 1950s, and more recent Australian studies, suggest important pre-eruptive benefits and support continuous exposure for the best outcome [5,7,10,11]. These investigators noted that a thin fluorapatite coating on the surface of hydroxyapatite crystals could lead to decreased solubility of enamel. Regardless of the predominant mechanism of action, water is an efficient vehicle for delivering a low concentration of fluoride at high frequency: that is, as it is consumed throughout the day.

Community water fluoridation

Fluoridation of community drinking water is the precise adjustment of the existing natural fluoride concentration in drinking water to a safe level that is recommended for caries prevention. The United States Public Health Service has established the optimum concentration for fluoride in the water in the range of 0.7 mg/L to 1.2 mg/L [12]. The optimum level for a region depends upon the annual average of the maximum daily air temperature. As of 2002, more than 170 million people in the United States, or 67% of those using public water supplies, drink water containing the recommended level of fluoride to prevent caries [13].

In the United States, 10 states have laws requiring communities to implement fluoridation if they meet certain conditions. In other states, the decision to fluoridate is usually made by individual communities. The water fluoridation program is usually administered under the supervision of state health and environmental agencies. Technical assistance is provided by the Division of Oral Health of the Centers for Disease Control and Prevention, whereas the Engineering and Administrative Recommendations for Water Fluoridation provides guidance for program administration [14].

Effectiveness of fluoridation

Early studies of water fluoridation suggested caries reductions in the range of 50% to 70% in children [15]. To test the relative effectiveness and cost of various interventions under modern conditions, the Robert Wood Johnson Foundation supported a large-scale study of school children in 10 different cities. This study showed that water fluoridation was the most cost-effective means of reducing tooth decay in children [16]. Fig. 1 compares the 4-year mean increment in caries between fluoridated and nonfluoridated communities among cohorts of fifth grade children that received class room and clinic interventions, and the cohort of longitudinal control groups receiving no intervention in fluoridated and nonfluoridated communities. Several recent authoritative reviews conducted in the United

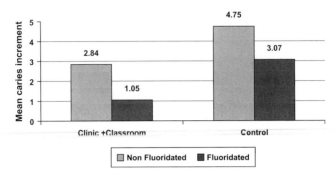

Fig. 1. Comparison of mean 4-year caries increment between intervention and control groups in fluoridated and nonfluoridated areas in cohorts of fifth grade children. Data for only four groups are presented. The classroom and clinic intervention included rinse (tablets in nonfluori-dated areas) plus lessons plus brushing plus sealants plus Prophy/Gel. (*Data from* Klein SP, Bohannan HM, Bell RM, Disney JA, Foch CB, Graves RC. The cost and effectiveness of school-based preventive dental care. Am J Public Health 1985;75(4):382–91.)

States, Australia, United Kingdom, and Ireland provide further evidence of the effectiveness of water fluoridation under conditions in which there is widespread exposure to fluoride from sources other than drinking water, such as fluoridated toothpastes and bottled beverages manufactured with fluoridated water [17–20]. The National Health Center for Reviews and Dissemination, University of York, concluded that the best available evidence suggested that fluoridation of drinking water supplies reduced dental caries prevalence, both as measured by the proportion of children who are caries-free and by the mean change in decayed, missing, and filled teeth score [17].

An independent Task Force convened by the Centers for Disease Control and Prevention that developed the *Guide to Community Preventive Services,* found strong evidence that water fluoridation is effective in reducing the cumulative caries experience in the population [18]. The Task Force computed estimates of effectiveness based on three groups of studies. In studies examining the before and after measurements of caries at the tooth level, starting or continuing fluoridation decreased dental caries experience among children aged 4 to 17 years by a median of 29.1% during 3 to 12 years of follow-up. In studies that examined only post exposure measurements of caries at the tooth level, starting or continuing fluoridation decreased dental caries experience among children aged 4 to 17 years by a median of 50.7% during 3 to 12 years of follow-up.

Fig. 2 shows several recent reports in the United States. The difference in dental caries between fluoridated and nonfluoridated communities is still noticeable, despite the ubiquitous presence of fluoride in food, water, and dental products [21–26]. Additional supportive evidence comes from studies conducted in Australia and Ireland [27–31].

In a United States national survey, the mean DMFS of 5- to 17-year-old children with continuous residence in fluoridated areas under modern

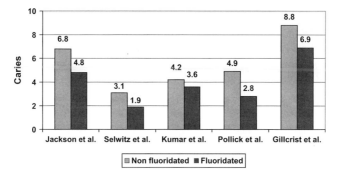

Fig. 2. Dental caries in fluoridated and nonfluoridated communities in studies conducted between 1995 and 2001. Jackson et al, mean DMFS in 11- to 14-year-old children; Selwitz et al, age adjusted mean DMFS in 8- to16-year-old children; Kumar et al, covariate adjusted mean DMFS plus dfs in second grade children; Pollick et al, covariate adjusted mean dfs in kindergarten to third grade children; Gillcrist et al, covariate adjusted mean dfs. (*Data from* Refs. [21–24,26]).

conditions of fluoride exposure was about 18% lower than in those with no exposure to fluoridation [32]. The availability of other forms of fluoride and the diffusion of fluoride through beverages and foods processed in fluoridated communities are thought to provide an explanation for the diminished difference in caries observed in recent years between fluoridated and nonfluoridated communities [32,33]. For example, children living in nonfluoridated areas in states such as Ohio, with more than 90% fluoridated areas, are more likely to receive the indirect benefit of water fluoridation through a diffusion effect (high diffusion) than that of in a state like New Jersey, where the fluoridation penetration is lower (low diffusion). According to Griffin and colleagues [34], on average, 12-year-old girls living in nonfluoridated areas with the least amount of exposure to a diffused effect experienced 1.44 more DMFS than did similar children residing in fluoridated communities. The indirect benefit of fluoridation, as evidenced by a comparison between children living in nonfluoridated communities with a high amount of fluoride exposure through diffusion and children living in nonfluoridated areas with the least amount of exposure to diffused effect, was an average of 1.09 fewer DMFS [33].

Cost effectiveness and cost savings

The National Preventive Dentistry Demonstration Program (NPDDP) reported that the reductions in decay attributable to water fluoridation were almost the same as those obtained with sealants [16]. These investigators estimated the costs of maintaining a child in a sealant program to be $23 per year, while the annual per capita cost of water fluoridation is substantially lower. Many factors, such as equipment, installation, chemicals, and labor, affect the cost of fluoridating a community [35]. The size of the community is a major determinant. According to the *Guide to Community Preventive Services*, the estimated median cost per person per year in the United States ranged from $2.70 for systems serving fewer than or equal to 5,000 people, to $0.40 for systems serving greater than or equal to 20,000 people [18].

Fluoridation has been shown to be cost saving. In 2001, Griffin and colleagues [35] estimated that for every one dollar expended, fluoridation saved $38 in treatment costs. Using similar methods, O'Connell and colleagues [36] estimated that the fluoridation program in Colorado was associated with an annual savings of $148.9 million (range, $115.1 to $187.2 million) in 2003, or an average of approximately $61 per person.

School-based fluoride mouth rinse programs

Fluoride mouth rinses were developed in the 1960s as an alternative to professional applications of gels and other topical fluoride products in school settings. With the availability of fluoridated water and fluoride con-taining toothpastes, these programs are now targeted to high-risk schools in nonfluoridated areas.

Typically, schools are provided with a year's supply of mouth rinse that consists of unit doses of 0.2% neutral sodium fluoride solutions in 5-mL or 10-mL pouches, along with cups and napkins. Children in grades one through six participate after obtaining written permission from parents. The procedure consists of vigorously rinsing with 5 mL or 10 mL of solution for 60 seconds on a weekly basis in the classroom under the supervision of a teacher, nurse, or a dental hygienist. After the rinsing, the fluoride solution is expectorated into a cup, a napkin is inserted into the cup to absorb the solution, and both are disposed. Younger children are provided with only 5 mL of solution. Fluoride mouth rinse programs are not recommended for preschool children in the United States, as some children may swallow the solution intended for topical application.

There are several advantages with the school-based fluoride rinse program. Generally, compliance is better because children perform the procedure as a group activity under supervision. Children tend to complain less about the taste when compared with that of topical fluorides. Because fluoride rinses are generally administered by volunteers, the cost per child is less when compared with that of professionally applied topical fluorides. However, the program requires trained personnel, a supervising dentist or registered dental hygienist, physician or nurse practitioner, and cooperation from teachers and school authorities.

Effectiveness

School-based fluoride mouth rinse programs have been the subject of nu-merous reviews [2,37,38]. A 17-site national school-based demonstration program showed that a protocol involving weekly rinsing with 0.2% sodium fluoride was a practical alternative to professional applications. Caries reductions ranging from 20% to 50% were observed. These estimates of caries reduction have been criticized because these programs relied on a before-and-after design, with no concurrent comparison group during a period of time when caries was declining in the United States. Analyses of the NPDDP data showed that dental health lessons, brushing and flossing, fluoride tablets and mouth rinsing, and professionally applied topical fluorides were not effective in reducing a substantial amount of dental decay, even when all of these procedures were used together [16]. Another study on the island of Guam, using a combination of sealant and fluoride mouth rinsing, showed a 25.4% caries reduction, mainly on the proximal surfaces with fluoride mouth rinsing [39]. Caries declined from 7.06 DMFS at the baseline to 2.93 DMFS after 10 years among 6- to 14-year-old children [39].

Cost-effectiveness

According to Garcia [40], the cost of the procedure in 1988 ranged between $0.52 and $1.78 per child per school year, depending on whether paid or volunteer adult supervisors were used. At present, the cost of the product to rinse weekly in a school for 36 weeks is approximately $2.64 per child. The NPDDP conducted during the late 1970s, when downward trends of caries rates were noted, questioned the cost-effectiveness of rinse programs [16]. Many experts have concluded that fluoride mouth rinses may be more cost-effective when targeted at schoolchildren with high caries activity [2,37]. Since then, many states, like New York, have targeted the fluoride rinse program to high-risk schools in nonfluoridated areas.

Fluoride tablet program

In tablet form, dietary fluoride supplements can be chewed and swallowed to provide topical and systemic fluoride for children in the absence of optimally fluoridated drinking water. A National Health Interview Survey found that some 16% of children younger than 2 years of age reportedly used dietary supplements [41]. Similar to school-based mouth rinse programs, fluoride tablet programs are structured as a group activity in settings such as Head Start centers. There are also programs designed to provide fluoride tablets to children of migrant farm workers. Generally, these programs target high-risk children in nonfluoridated areas.

The fluoride supplement dosage schedule developed by the American Dental Association [42] is based on the level of fluoride in the community water supply and on the age of the child (Table 2). Fluoride supplements, however, should not be prescribed for individuals in communities where fluoride has been adjusted to optimal levels in the water or in places where optimal amounts of fluoride occur naturally in drinking water.

Table 2
Dietary fluoride supplement dosage schedule

Age of child	Fluoride dosage (milligrams per day) at fluoride in water concentration of:		
	< 0.3 ppm	0.3 ppm to 0.6 ppm	> 0.6 ppm
Birth to 6 months	None	None	None
6 months to 3 years	0.25	None	None
3–6 years	0.50	0.25	None
6–16 years	1.00	0.50	None

Data from American Dental Association. Council on access prevention and interpersonal relations. Caries diagnosis and risk assessment: a review of preventive strategies and management. J Am Dent Assoc 1995;126:S2–24z.

Effectiveness

Fluoride tablet programs in schools have been shown to be effective in preventing caries in permanent teeth when children are instructed to let the tablet dissolve slowly, to ensure as much topical fluoride exposure as possible. Under these conditions, randomized controlled trials in the United States reported caries reductions of 20% to 28% over periods of 3 to 6 years [43,44]. In a randomized, double-blind, 3-year study of Scottish schoolchildren who were 5.5 years of age at the start of the study, an 81% reduction in caries in permanent teeth was observed [45,46]. In this study, teachers were specifically requested to encourage children each school day to let the sodium fluoride tablet dissolve slowly. These children were likely at high risk for dental caries, because they were from lower socio-economic groups and may not have had access to fluoride-containing dentifrices. According to the Centers for Disease Control [12], while the evidence for school based fluoride supplement programs for 6 to 16 year olds is strong, the quality of the evidence for programs in younger children is weak.

Cost-effectiveness

According to the Surgeon General's report: Oral Health in America [2], school-based tablet programs have low costs because equipment is not necessary, the procedure does not take long, and an entire classroom of children can participate at once. In 1989, Garcia [40] found an average direct cost of approximately $2.53 per child per school year. While economic benefits of a fluoride supplement program in Manchester, England, showed overall health and cost benefits [46], an earlier study in the United States did not find fluoride supplements to be cost effective in a school-based program [14].

School-based fluoride tablet programs are likely to be effective in providing topical fluoride protection for children at high risk for dental caries in settings where supervising personnel are highly motivated [47,48]. Under these conditions, such programs may also be cost-effective [2].

Supervised tooth brushing programs with fluoridated toothpaste

In a supervised tooth brushing program, brushing is conducted once each day in the classroom or in Head Start centers using a fluoridated toothpaste. Teachers or other volunteers that are trained in an appropriate tooth brushing technique supervise the administration of the program. It requires trained personnel to ensure proper labeling and storage of toothbrushes. Two to four children are brought to a sink and a pea-sized amount of toothpaste is dispensed on the back of a paper cup by a Head Start staff or a classroom teacher. Children are instructed to brush for 1 minute and spit. In addition to the costs of the toothpaste and toothbrushes, the difficulty of storing toothbrushes and the labor-intensive nature of the program may be barriers for some sites.

Effectiveness

A systematic review of 70 controlled clinical trials of fluoridated toothpastes found that a greater amount of dental caries was prevented when tooth brushing was supervised [49]. This observation underscores the concept that the benefits of fluoridated toothpaste can be enhanced by structuring the environment to assure that children are brushing their teeth on a regular basis, and that this habit is instilled for a lifelong healthy behavior.

A 2-year clinical trial of supervised tooth brushing in 5 year olds found a 32% reduction in caries increment attributable to the intervention in Scotland [50]. Similarly, an evaluation of a supervised tooth brushing program for 5 and 6 year olds in England found an 11% reduction in caries increment [51].

Cost-effectiveness

Data are not available on cost-effectiveness associated with supervised tooth brushing programs.

Fluoride varnish programs

Fluoride varnishes have been available as anticaries agents in Europe and Canada for over two decades. In the United States, it has been approved for use as a desensitizing agent. The varnishes are painted onto teeth and provide a reservoir of fluoride that is released over time in close proximity to the enamel surface. While fluoride retention from varnishes is greater than with solutions or gels, the varnishes must be reapplied by a professional to maintain their cariostatic effect. Recently, the American Dental Association Council on Scientific Affairs [52] summarized evidence and concluded that fluoride varnish applied every 6 months is effective in preventing caries in primary and permanent teeth of children and adolescents at risk for caries.

Fluoride varnish is attractive in a public health program because it can be easily incorporated into well-child visits to control early childhood caries. Innovative programs involving the application of fluoride varnish by physicians, nurses, and other health professionals to children have been initiated in many states. The North Carolina oral screening and fluoride varnish project, called "Into the Mouths of Babes," is a collaborative effort among several partners [53]. The objective of the program is to train medical providers to deliver preventive oral health services to high-risk children from the time of tooth eruption until the third birthday. The preventive procedure consists of oral screening, individualized face-to-face parent or caregiver education, and application of fluoride varnish. Other states, such as Minnesota, Virginia, and Michigan have also developed programs to target Head Start children.

Effectiveness

Research on the effectiveness and costs associated with community-based fluoride varnish programs for high risk groups is ongoing. In the United States, a clinical trial conducted in young children showed that fluoride varnish was effective in reducing caries [54]. A meta-analysis conducted by Marinho and colleagues [55] showed that fluoride varnish could reduce caries in primary dentition by approximately one third.

Cost-effectiveness

The cost of application of fluoride varnish has been estimated to be in the range of $16 to $19 per application. A simulated analysis showed that fluoride varnish in the medical setting is effective in reducing early childhood caries in low-income populations, but is not cost saving in the first 42 months of life [56]. This can be attributed to the relatively low incidence of caries in this age group. The early intervention may yield cost savings in later years as children grow older and their risk for developing caries increases.

Salt fluoridation

Salt fluoridation is the controlled addition of fluoride to domestic salt for purposes of preventing dental caries. Similar to water fluoridation, a small amount of fluoride is widely distributed to the population in salt that is consumed on a daily basis. Like water fluoridation, salt fluoridation requires little effort on the consumer's part.

Salt fluoridation is attractive where water supplies are low in fluoride. Switzerland, Colombia, Hungary, Costa Rica, Jamaica, and Mexico have all had considerable experience with salt fluoridation. It is estimated that 150 million individuals world-wide use fluoridated domestic salt (80 million in Europe, 70 million in Latin America and the Caribbean) [57].

Effectiveness

Community trials in Colombia and Hungary were conducted beginning in the 1960s to determine the effectiveness of salt fluoridation in preventing dental caries. These studies showed the reduction in dental caries prevalence to be about 50% in communities that had salt fluoridation programs [58]. These findings provide evidence that salt fluoridation reduced caries levels to an extent similar to water fluoridation.

Cost-effectiveness and cost savings

The cost of salt fluoridation has been estimated that for every dollar spent on salt fluoridation, about $250 in dental treatment costs are saved, making salt fluoridation an attractive public health investment [58].

Policy considerations

Public health policies should be based on sound science about risks, benefits, and economic evaluation of interventions to address a specific problem in a community. Decision makers should also consider the impact of not implementing a proven intervention. According to Brownson and colleagues [59], the control of chronic diseases is most effective if environmental and policy approaches are the earliest focus of change. Because individual behaviors are difficult to change in those who are especially at high risk, public health practitioners promote changes in the environment that benefit everyone. Some recent examples include the addition of folic acid to food grains to prevent neural tube defects, laws to prohibit smoking in public places, and restriction on the use of oils containing trans fats for cooking.

In the United States, water fluoridation is considered the cornerstone of a sound public health practice. Water fluoridation creates an environment conducive to promoting good oral health. Fluoridation delivers a sustainable level of fluoride to the oral environment on a frequent basis in an inexpensive way. It is a low-cost intervention that can reach large populations without active participation of the individuals. It provides preventive benefit across the spectrum of low and high socio-economic groups and may reduce disparities in oral health. Therefore, Healthy People 2010, a set of national objectives, has set a national goal of reaching 75% of the population on public water supplies. To reach this goal, the number of people on fluoridation should increase from 170 million to approximately 185 million.

The science based on effectiveness, safety, and the benefits of water fluoridation is extensive. It has been practiced in many countries for well over 50 years. In communicating the risks associated with water fluoridation, it is important to inform the community that benefits outweigh the risks. The only risk associated with the ingestion of fluoridated water at optimal levels is the occurrence of milder forms of enamel fluorosis [17]. In the United States, the decline in dental caries has also been accompanied by an increase in the prevalence of enamel fluorosis, both in fluoridated and nonfluoridated communities [60]. Undoubtedly, sources such as fluoride toothpaste ingestion during the development of teeth, and inappropriate use of fluoride supplements, have contributed to the excessive intake. Therefore, several steps have been taken to reduce fluoride exposure from various sources. These include a reduction in the fluoride content in infant formulas, revision of the fluoride supplement schedule, and recommendations to lower fluoride exposure from toothpastes for children under age 6 [12].

Discussions about fluoridation of a particular community should focus on the disease burden, feasibility, cost, and use of other forms of fluoride. Decision makers should be made aware of the benefits and risks. While exposure to fluoridation and daily use of fluoride toothpaste is sufficient for most Americans, some individuals may need additional targeted interventions. In areas where fluoridation is not available, an alternative public health program may be considered.

Summary

The use of fluorides in dental public health programs has a long history. With the availability of fluoridation and other forms of fluorides, dental caries has declined dramatically in the United States. Fluoride acts both topically after the eruption of teeth and systemically through its incorporation into enamel crystals. The science based on effectiveness, safety, and the benefits of water fluoridation and other forms of fluoride is extensive. For most people, fluoride exposure through water fluoridation and regular tooth brushing is sufficient. Routine application of topical gels or foams for 1 minute is no longer supported by evidence. Populations at high risk may need additional exposure through other forms of fluorides. In areas where fluoridation is not available, an alternative public health program may be considered.

References

[1] Beltran-Aguilar ED, Barker LK, Canto MT, et al. Surveillance for dental caries, dental sealants, tooth retention, edentulism, and enamel fluorosis—United States, 1988–1994 and 1999–2002. MMWR Surveill Summ 2005;54(3):1–43.
[2] US Department of Health and Human Services. Oral health in America: A Report of the Surgeon General. Rockville (MD): National Institute of Health; 2000.
[3] McClure FJ. Fluorine in drinking waters. US Department of Health, Education, and Welfare. Bethesda (MD): Public Health Service, National Institute of Dental Research; 1962.
[4] Burt BA, Eklund SA. Dentistry, dental practice and the community. 6th edition. Missouri (MO): Elsevier Saunders; 2005.
[5] Arnold FA Jr. Grand Rapids fluoridation study; results pertaining to the eleventh year of fluoridation. Am J Public Health Nations Health 1957;47(5):539–45.
[6] Arnold FA. The use of fluorides in the practice of dental medicine. Oral Surg Oral Med Oral Pathol 1950;3(5):622–30.

[7] Ast DB, Smith DJ, Wachs B, et al. Newburgh-Kingston caries-fluorine study. XIV. Combined clinical and roentgenographic dental findings after ten years of fluoride experience. J Am Dent Assoc 1956;52(3):314–25.

[8] Featherstone JD. Prevention and reversal of dental caries: role of low level fluoride. Community Dent Oral Epidemiol 1999;27(1):31–40.

[9] Featherstone JD. The science and practice of caries prevention. J Am Dent Assoc 2000; 131(7):887–99.

[10] Singh KA, Spencer AJ, Armfield JM. Relative effects of pre- and posteruption water fluoride on caries experience of permanent first molars. J Public Health Dent 2003;63(1):11–9.

[11] Singh KA, Spencer AJ. Relative effects of pre- and post-eruption water fluoride on caries experience by surface type of permanent first molars. Community Dent Oral Epidemiol 2004; 32(6):435–46.

[12] Centers for Disease Control and Prevention. Recommendations for using fluoride to prevent and control dental caries in the United States. MMWR Recomm Rep 2001;50(RR-14): 1–30.

[13] Centers for Disease Control and Prevention. Background information. Available at: http://www.cdc.gov/fluoridation/benefits/background.htm. Accessed September 25, 2007.

[14] Centers for Disease Control and Prevention. Engineering and administrative recommendations for water fluoridation. MMWR Recomm Rep 1995;29:1–40.

[15] Centers for Disease Control and Prevention. Achievements in public health, 1900–1999: fluoridation of drinking water to prevent dental caries. MMWR 1999;48(41):933–40.

[16] Klein SP, Bohannan HM, Bell RM, et al. The cost and effectiveness of school-based preventive dental care. Am J Public Health 1985;75(4):382–91.

[17] McDonagh MS, Whiting PF, Wilson PM, et al. Systematic review of water fluoridation. BMJ 2000;321(7265):855–9.

[18] Truman BI, Gooch BF, Sulemana I, et al. Reviews of evidence on interventions to prevent dental caries, oral and pharyngeal cancers, and sports-related craniofacial injuries. Am J Prev Med 2002;23(1 Suppl):21–54.

[19] Government of Ireland. Forum on Fluoridation. Dublin (Ireland): Government of Ireland; 2002. p. 1–296.

[20] National Health and Medical Research Council. A systematic review of the efficacy and safety of fluoridation. Canberra, Australia: 2007.

[21] Jackson RD, Kelly SA, Katz BP, et al. Dental fluorosis and caries prevalence in children residing in communities with different levels of fluoride in the water. J Public Health Dent 1995; 55(2):79–84.

[22] Gillcrist JA, Brumley DE, Blackford JU. Community fluoridation status and caries experience in children. J Public Health Dent 2001;61(3):168–71.

[23] Kumar JV, Green EL, Coluccio C, et al. Oral health status of second grade school children in upstate New York. NY State Dent J 2001;67(2):26–31.

[24] Selwitz RH, Nowjack-Raymer RE, Kingman A, et al. Prevalence of dental caries and dental fluorosis in areas with optimal and above-optimal water fluoride concentrations: a 10-year follow-up survey. J Public Health Dent 1995;55(2):85–93.

[25] Selwitz RH, Nowjack-Raymer RE, Kingman A, et al. Dental caries and dental fluorosis among schoolchildren who were lifelong residents of communities having either low or optimal levels of fluoride in drinking water. J Public Health Dent 1998;58(1):28–35.

[26] Pollick HF, Isman R, Fine JI, et al. Report of the California oral health needs assessment of children, 1993–94: background, methodology, findings. Oakland (California): The Dental Health Foundation; 1999.

[27] Armfield JM. Public water fluoridation and dental health in New South Wales. Aust NZ J Public Health 2005;29(5):477–83.

[28] Hopcraft MS, Morgan MV. Exposure to fluoridated drinking water and dental caries experience in Australian army recruits, 1996. Community Dent Oral Epidemiol 2003;31(1): 68–74.

[29] Hopcraft MS, Morgan MV. Comparison of radiographic and clinical diagnosis of approximal and occlusal dental caries in a young adult population. Community Dent Oral Epidemiol 2005;33(3):212–8.

[30] Slade GD, Davies MJ, Spencer AJ, et al. Associations between exposure to fluoridated drinking water and dental caries experience among children in two Australian states. J Public Health Dent 1995;55(4):218–28.

[31] Slade GD, Spencer AJ, Davies MJ, et al. Influence of exposure to fluoridated water on socioeconomic inequalities in children's caries experience. Community Dent Oral Epidemiol 1996;24(2):89–100.

[32] Brunelle JA, Carlos JP. Recent trends in dental caries in U.S. children and the effect of water fluoridation. J Dent Res 1990;69(3pec No):723–7.

[33] Ripa LW. A half-century of community water fluoridation in the United States: review and commentary. J Public Health Dent 1993;53(1):17–44.

[34] Griffin SO, Gooch BF, Lockwood SA, et al. Quantifying the diffused benefit from water fluoridation in the United States. Community Dent Oral Epidemiol 2001;29(2):120–9.

[35] Griffin SO, Jones K, Tomar SL. An economic evaluation of community water fluoridation. J Public Health Dent 2001;61(2):78–86.

[36] O'Connell JM, Brunson D, Anselmo T, et al. Costs and savings associated with community water fluoridation programs in Colorado. Prev Chronic Dis 2005;2:1–13.

[37] Leverett DH. Effectiveness of mouthrinsing with fluoride solutions in preventing coronal and root caries. J Public Health Dent 1989;49(5 Spec No):310–6.

[38] Stamm JW, Bohannan HM, Graves RC, et al. The efficiency of caries prevention with weekly fluoride mouthrinses. J Dent Educ 1984;48(11):617–26.

[39] Sterritt GR, Frew RA, Rozier RG. Evaluation of Guamanian dental caries preventive programs after 13 years. J Public Health Dent 1994;54(3):153–9.

[40] Garcia AI. Caries incidence and costs of prevention programs. J Public Health Dent 1989; 49(5 Spec No):259–71.

[41] Nourjah P, Horowitz AM, Wagener DK. Factors associated with the use of fluoride supplements and fluoride dentifrice by infants and toddlers. J Public Health Dent 1994;54(1):47–54.

[42] American Dental Association. Council on Access Prevention and Interpersonal Relations. Caries diagnosis and risk assessment: a review of preventive strategies and management. J Am Dent Assoc 1995;126:S2–24.

[43] DePaola PF, Lax M. The caries-inhibiting effect of acidulated phosphate-fluoride chewable tablets: a two-year double-blind study. J Am Dent Assoc 1968;76(3):554–7.

[44] Driscoll WS, Heifetz SB, Korts DC. Effect of chewable fluoride tablets on dental caries in schoolchildren: results after six years of use. J Am Dent Assoc 1978;97(5):820–4.

[45] Stephen KW, Campbell D. Caries reduction and cost benefit after 3 years of sucking fluoride tablets daily at school. A double-blind trial. Br Dent J 1978;144(7):202–6.

[46] O'Rourke CA, Attrill M, Holloway PJ. Cost appraisal of a fluoride tablet programme to Manchester primary schoolchildren. Community Dent Oral Epidemiol 1988;16(6):341–4.

[47] Clarkson J. A European view of fluoride supplementation. Br Dent J 1992;172(9):357.

[48] Ismail AI. Fluoride supplements: current effectiveness, side effects, and recommendations. Community Dent Oral Epidemiol 1994;22(3):164–72.

[49] Marinho VC, Higgins JP, Sheiham A, et al. Fluoride toothpastes for preventing dental caries in children and adolescents. Cochrane Database Syst Rev 2003;(1):CD002278.

[50] Curnow MM, Pine CM, Burnside G, et al. A randomised controlled trial of the efficacy of supervised toothbrushing in high-caries-risk children. Caries Res 2002;36(4):294–300.

[51] Jackson RJ, Newman HN, Smart GJ, et al. The effects of a supervised toothbrushing programme on the caries increment of primary school children, initially aged 5–6 years. Caries Res 2005;39(2):108–15.

[52] ADA. Council on Scientific Affairs. Professionally applied topical fluoride: evidence-based clinical recommendations. J Am Dent Assoc 2006;137(8):1151–9.

[53] Rozier RG, Sutton BK, Bawden JW, et al. Prevention of early childhood caries in North Carolina medical practices: implications for research and practice. J Dent Educ 2003;67(8):876–85.

[54] Weintraub JA, Ramos-Gomez F, Jue B, et al. Fluoride varnish efficacy in preventing early childhood caries. J Dent Res 2006;85(2):172–6.

[55] Marinho VC, Higgins IP, Logan S, et al. Fluoride varnishes for preventing dental caries in children and adolescents. Cochrane Database Syst Rev 2002;(3):CD002279.

[56] Quinonez RB, Stearns SC, Talekar BS, et al. Simulating cost-effectiveness of fluoride varnish during well-child visits for Medicaid-enrolled children. Arch Pediatr Adolesc Med 2006; 160(2):164–70.

[57] Estupinan-Day S. Promoting oral health: the use of salt fluoridation to prevent dental caries. Washington, DC: Pan American Health Organization; 2005.

[58] Estupinan-Day SR, Baez R, Horowitz H, et al. Salt fluoridation and dental caries in Jamaica. Community Dent Oral Epidemiol 2001;29(4):247–52.

[59] Brownson RC, Haire-Joshu D, Luke DA. Shaping the context of health: a review of environmental and policy approaches in the prevention of chronic diseases. Annu Rev Public Health 2006;27:341–70.

[60] Rozier RG. The prevalence and severity of enamel fluorosis in North American children. J Public Health Dent 1999;59(4):239–46.

ELSEVIER
SAUNDERS

THE DENTAL
CLINICS
OF NORTH AMERICA

Dent Clin N Am 52 (2008) 403–421

Planning and Evaluating Community Oral Health Programs

Scott L. Tomar, DMD, DrPH

*Department of Community Dentistry and Behavioral Science, University of Florida College
of Dentistry, 1329 SW 16th Street, PO Box 103628, Gainesville, FL 32610–3628, USA*

Community oral health programs

Dentistry traditionally has focused primarily on providing care to individual patients on a one-on-one basis. Most United States residents seek dental care from dentists in private practice, who diagnose disease, develop a treatment plan, and provide care. This model of care works reasonably well for much of the public but has several key deficiencies:

- There are financial, geographic, cultural, attitudinal, and other barriers that restrict access to private practice- based dental care for a large segment of the public;
- Despite policy statements and recommendations from organizations such as the American Academy of Pediatric Dentistry [1], preventive dental visits remain very rare among young children. It remains uncertain whether there is adequate capacity in the United States to provide dental care for all children by 12 months of age [2];
- Prevention services often can be delivered in a more cost-effective manner in venues other than private dental offices;
- Dental public health problems frequently require policy initiatives, community-based initiatives, and environmental changes that are outside the scope of the individual private practice dental office.

Population versus individual approach

There are several key differences between a personal dental care approach and a community oral health approach to controlling oral disease in a population. Personal dental care requires an individual to visit a dentist, who then initiates care by taking a dental and medical history and conducting

---

E-mail address: stomar@dental.ufl.edu

an examination. The dentist arrives at a diagnosis and develops a treatment plan. After obtaining the patient's informed consent, the dentist renders dental care, collects his or her fee, and schedules the patient for a follow-up visit.

Community oral health programs follow steps analogous to those taken by an individual dentist but focus primarily on a population, including persons who do not or cannot access care, rather than just one patient in the chair. The director of a community oral health program collects the necessary information to identify community problems, much like an individual dentist diagnoses a patient's condition. The director then uses that information to develop policies and programs to address the problem, just as the individual dentist develops a treatment plan. Finally, the community oral health program delivers services to the community, as a dentist would provide treatment. Those services likely include more than provision of patient-based clinical care.

Reach versus intensity

Because dental public health is focused on the oral health of communities and populations and always operates within the constraints of financing and feasibility, the types of services provided involve a balance between what might work best for an individual and what might be possible to deliver to entire populations. Often, programs that reach a wider audience but are less intensive for any one person—and therefore perhaps less effective at an individual level—may produce better population health outcomes than far more intensive interventions delivered to a much smaller group.

For example, intensive smoking cessation treatments, such as group behavior therapy programs, are more effective than self-help alone [3], but because so few smokers are willing to participate in such intensive programs, they will have almost no measurable effect in reducing the prevalence of smoking in a population. In comparison, weaker and relatively inexpensive interventions, such as increasing the cost of cigarettes through taxation and changing the environmental norm through workplace smoking restrictions, can lead to large reductions in smoking and, consequently, fewer smoking-related deaths [4].

Similar effects are possible with dental caries prevention programs. For example, community water fluoridation may have lower effectiveness than twice-a-year applications of fluoride varnish by a dental hygienist for an individual at high risk for caries [5,6], but water fluoridation may likely prevent much more disease in a population because of its reach.

Balancing individual rights and societal protection

Public health practice, particularly in the United States, frequently involves a contentious balance between individual rights and societal benefit.

Motorcycle helmet laws typify this tension: despite overwhelming epidemiologic evidence that motorcycle helmets reduce fatalities and serious injuries, many motorcycle riders perceive such laws as an infringement on personal liberties [7]. Proponents of motorcycle helmet laws argue that a burden is placed on society when an individual suffers injury or death from preventable motorcycle fatalities [8]. Similar arguments of individual rights versus social good have been made regarding dental public health policies including, for example, community water fluoridation [9] and school-based dental screening [10].

Planning and evaluating community oral health programs

Planning may be defined as a systematic approach to defining a problem, setting priorities, developing specific goals and objectives, and determining alternative strategies and methods of implementation [11]. Although typically described as a linear series of steps or as a cyclical process (Fig. 1), program planning usually involves an ongoing, dynamic process with multiple interactions among the components. So, although the process is described as a series of steps, many of the activities involved in planning and evaluation can occur simultaneously or involve modifications along the way. For example, assessment of needs and resources can occur simultaneously, and the process of setting goals and objectives frequently involves reassessing the available resources to determine the feasibility of pursuing some program objectives.

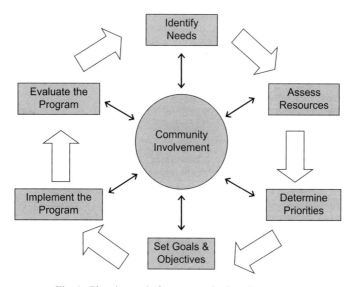

Fig. 1. Planning cycle for community-based programs.

Although there are many textbooks, book chapters, and journal articles on program planning, relatively few focus specifically on community oral health programs. The framework below draws on the expertise and experiences of state and local dental program directors, academicians, and organizations, as captured in "A Guide for Developing and Enhancing Community Oral Health Programs" [12].

Engage the community

A major key to successful community oral health program planning and implementation is involving community stakeholders in the process [13]. Community organizations, leaders, and institutions should be engaged as coalition members and partners as early as possible in the planning process.

A coalition is a group of diverse individuals and organizations who work together to achieve a common goal. Participants usually represent key organizations or groups within the community. These individuals meet regularly to exchange ideas, reach a common goal, and create a group dedicated to improving the lives of community members around a particular issue.

Oral health coalitions provide several major advantages: (1) they help highlight the importance and magnitude of oral health needs in the community; (2) they leverage support from multiple organizations and individuals to increase the resources available to address oral health issues; (3) they involve community organizations in planning to help ensure that programs will be feasible and culturally acceptable to the community; (4) they help increase trust among groups; and (5) initiatives endorsed and supported by a broad range of groups are more likely than solo efforts to garner attention and support from elected officials and policymakers, who can help secure resources and policy changes to reach program objectives.

Although governmental dental public health authorities have a unique responsibility to promote and protect the oral health of the people, growing realization that government cannot do it alone has led to calls for increasing public-private collaborations [14]. Public resources are always limited, and public health is just one of many societal priorities. The factors that impact public health come from a variety of sources and sectors, including employment, education, laws and policies, and social norms. Those sectors may need to be engaged in efforts to promote public health. There is a growing recognition that individuals, communities, and social institutions can form powerful collaborative relationships to improve health in ways that government alone cannot.

A partial list of potential coalition partners might include:

- Parent-teacher organizations
- Local chapters of professional groups, such as dental societies, dental hygiene associations, and primary care organizations
- Agencies that work with special needs populations, such individuals with disabilities

- Dental schools and dental hygiene programs
- Faith-based organizations
- Children's health advocacy groups
- Service organizations for older adults

Identify oral health needs

Before launching an oral health program, it is essential to first assess the oral health status and needs of the community. Data needed to plan, monitor, and evaluate dental public health policies and programs come from a number of sources. Although national and state-level data may exist, it is almost always preferable to plan and evaluate using local or community-level data. There are a variety of sources for such data, which may be readily available or require original data collection.

Sociodemographic characteristics of the community

A wide range of information at the county or local level is available from the US Census Bureau. For example, the decennial census and periodic surveys, such as the American Community Survey [15], provide data on characteristics of the county or city such as age, race, ethnicity, housing units, educational attainment, household income, and poverty status. Data for a number of characteristics are available for geographic areas smaller than counties, such as census tracts, block groups, or blocks.

Water fluoridation status

Information on the community water fluoridation status of nearly all public water systems in the United States is available from the Centers for Disease Control and Prevention (CDC), Division of Oral Health, at http://apps.nccd.cdc.gov/MWF/Index.asp. The information is updated periodically based on monitoring data submitted to the Water Fluoridation Reporting System. Access to the original data can be requested from individual state oral health programs and tribes.

Cancer registries

State-based cancer registries are data systems that collect, manage, and analyze data about cancer cases and cancer deaths. In each state, health care facilities report these data to a central cancer registry. These cancer registries provide the ability to monitor trends in the number of new cases of oral cancer, oral cancer incidence rates (ie, number of new cases per 100,000 population), oral cancer survival rates, and cancer stage at the time of diagnosis. These statistics are available for the total population within each state, as well as by sex, age, and race, at http://apps.nccd.cdc.gov/uscs.

Cancer registries can usually provide oral cancer data for counties or cities, which is useful in targeting areas with unusually high rates of new cases or late-stage diagnosis. For example, analysis of cancer registry data in

Florida helped to identify a multicounty area in the northeastern part of the state in which black males experienced a particularly high incidence rate (Fig. 2), which led to the development of a local oral cancer awareness and screening program.

Clinical surveys

At least 15 state dental programs have conducted statewide clinical surveys within the past six years, although none included adults [16]. Most states employed the Basic Screening Survey (BSS), which was developed by the Association of State and Territorial Dental Directors [17]. The BSS was developed as a simple training and data collection tool that could be used by screeners with or without dental backgrounds. That approach was taken because nondental health professionals, such as public health nurses, sometimes have direct access to some population groups and because some states and communities have few public health dental professionals to assist in screening surveys. The BSS has components for collecting clinical oral health data for preschool-aged children, school children, and adults.

The primary barriers to collection of original clinical data are expense and logistic difficulties. Clinical surveys often require training personnel to conduct the examinations, traveling to multiple locations, obtaining portable or mobile dental equipment, adhering to infection control protocols, and gaining the cooperation and trust of school officials, parents, and children. Clinical surveys of adults are particularly difficult and expensive, which

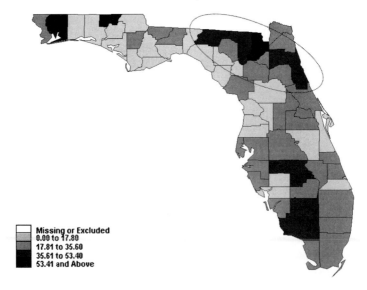

Missing or Excluded
0.00 to 17.80
17.81 to 35.60
35.61 to 53.40
53.41 and Above

Fig. 2. Oral cancer incidence rate for black males in Florida, 1990–1999 combined, by county, age-adjusted to the 2000 U.S. standard population. Oval indicates area with high incidence targeted for intervention program. (*Data from* the Florida Cancer Data System.)

explains in part why there are almost no clinical data on adult oral health at the state or local levels.

Nonclinical oral health surveys

A good deal of information relevant to planning and evaluating oral health issues can be obtained from nonclinical surveys. These surveys involve collection of data via telephone, face-to-face interviews, or self-completed questionnaires but do not require clinical examination of participants. These types of surveys are often the most economically and logistically feasible ways to reach adults. Valid data on many relevant oral health topics can be covered through self-reported surveys.

One relatively cost-effective approach for gathering oral health-related data at the state, county, or local level is to partner with other organizations or agencies that will be conducting surveys and add relevant oral health questions. For example, the Behavioral Risk Factor Surveillance System (BRFSS) is a state-based, ongoing telephone survey on preventive health practices and risk behaviors that are linked to chronic diseases, injuries, and preventable infectious diseases [18]. The BRFSS is administered in all states and the District of Columbia. All states include a core set of questions developed in conjunction with the CDC, several optional modules on a wide range of health topics, and a number of state-added questions. The BRFSS core questionnaire includes several oral health variables, including tooth loss, last dental visit, preventive care, and risk factors relevant to oral health. States frequently make their state-added questions available to groups working on health-related topics. States usually charge a fee per question added, but the cost is far less than that of a typical stand-alone telephone survey. A number of states periodically conduct county BRFSS surveys, in which the sample design allows estimates at the county level. Information on the BRFSS surveys is available at http://www.cdc.gov/brfss.

Health care providers, facilities, and programs

Information on the number and locations of area dentists, dental hygienists, and other licensed health care providers can usually be obtained from the state licensing authority. County and local dental societies also may be able to provide information on the number and location of dental specialists. The state government agency that oversees labor and employment frequently has data on the number and location of dental offices, clinics, and other health care facilities. Information on the number of providers participating in Medicaid or the State Children's Health Insurance Program (SCHIP) is available at the state agency that oversees those programs. The Health Resources and Services Administration, Bureau of Health Professions (HRSA-BHP) has information on the criteria and application process for designation as a dental health professional shortage area (HPSA). HRSA-BHP offers a searchable database of HPSAs with information available at the state, county, and census tract levels.

Putting it together

Even the best data are meaningless unless they can be analyzed and interpreted. When planning to assemble existing information or collect original data, it is critical to identify the individuals or organizations that will help with those tasks. Expertise may reside in the local or state health department, the nearby dental school or school of public health, or consultants. Coalition members may be able to offer such services as part of their contribution to the program or identify expertise elsewhere.

Assess resources

As mentioned earlier, one major benefit of forming a community oral health coalition is to leverage resources. Although any one organization may lack the resources to address major oral health problems by itself, a collaborative effort may pool the limited resources from multiple parties to be able to achieve a common goal.

Resources may include expertise, funding, personnel, equipment, or access to other influential individuals and organizations. It is not possible to list all potential resources, but some sources to consider include:

Dental schools, dental hygiene programs, and dental assisting programs

These institutions may be able to provide expertise and assistance in collection of oral health data, delivery of prevention or treatment services, and access to portable or mobile dental equipment. In addition, faculty may be able to serve as expert speakers on oral health topics. Most universities have communications offices, which may be able to help promote the program if their faculty members are involved in the project.

Schools of public health

Schools of public health can provide assistance with design and conduct of surveys and data analysis. In addition, many schools of public health have established community links and may be able to facilitate connections with community leaders and organizations. Students in schools of public health frequently need to complete internships or research projects, and their participation in community oral health programs can be mutually beneficial.

Federally qualified community health centers

Federally qualified community health centers, or FQHCs, are nonprofit, consumer-directed corporations that serve as "safety net" providers, such as community health centers, public housing centers, outpatient health programs funded by the Indian Health Service, and programs serving migrants and the homeless [19]. The main purpose of FQHCs is to enhance the provision of primary care services in underserved urban and rural communities. Most FQHCs provide dental services [20]. These health centers may be able to assist with expertise, program implementation, and access to community boards of directors.

Area health education centers

The Area Health Education Centers (AHEC) program was developed by Congress in 1971 to recruit, train, and retain a health professionals workforce committed to underserved populations [21]. The Health Education Training Centers (HETC) program was created in 1989 to provide programs for specific populations with persistent, severe, and unmet health needs. The AHEC and HETC programs are intended to leverage the resources of academic health centers to help address local community health needs. These programs can contribute substantial expertise and support in bringing dental students, residents, and faculty into underserved communities; developing and implementing service learning; and providing community education and wellness programs.

School nurses

Schools have long been major venues for reaching children to monitor oral health status and to deliver prevention and treatment services. Although not all schools have a nurse, school nurses play a vital role in ensuring the health of students, identifying health needs, and advocating for necessary resources. They can be a valuable resource in understanding the impact of oral health problems on learning, gathering data on the health status of the student population, and supporting delivery of oral health services in schools.

State and local dentistry and dental hygiene societies

Organized dentistry and dental hygiene societies can be critical resources in establishing dental public health programs. They bring a great deal of expertise to the process, and commitment from these organizations may be critical to long-term success.

Determine priorities and establish objectives

Setting priorities

Determining health priorities helps direct resources to the areas that matter most to community partners and that will have the greatest impact on oral health status. Few public health programs have the resources to address all oral health needs of the community. Therefore, after identifying the community's oral health needs and assessing the available resources, it is necessary to establish priorities. The community should be involved in establishing those priorities, and the problem of greatest interest to the health professionals in the coalition may not necessarily be the priority of the community members. Some of the factors to consider in prioritizing needs may include:

The magnitude and seriousness of the problem. Problems that affect a large number of people may take priority over problems that affect a small number. However, the relative prevalence of various conditions must be balanced against the severity and impact of those conditions. A widespread condition with minimal impact on health or quality of life may have a lower priority than a less common condition that carries a risk of fatality if not prevented or controlled or significantly impacts on quality of life for those affected. For example, gingivitis may have a very high prevalence, but might be considered a much lower priority than addressing late-stage diagnosis of oral and pharyngeal cancer.

The potential for interventions to impact the public's oral health. Ideally, there should be an evidence base indicating that there is an effective intervention for the problem. Spending resources on unproven preventive strategies or treatments may be wasteful.

The feasibility of intervening. In addition, possible interventions must be acceptable to the community, able to be delivered using available resources, and in compliance with state and local laws and regulations.

Developing program goals and objectives

Program goals are broad statements on the overall purpose of a program. Goals generally express the aspirations of the planners of the state of affairs that will exist in the future because of their efforts. Example of program goals might be "to eliminate racial disparities in oral cancer survival rates," "to improve the oral health of nursing home residents," or "to improve the oral health of the county's toddlers and school children."

Program objectives are more specific statements of the desired endpoints of the project. They are the means through which the project's broader goals are attained. As with other elements of the planning process, the objectives must represent the input and agreement of all members of the oral health coalition. Objectives for designing and evaluating community oral health programs should meet basic SMART criteria [22]:

Specific – they should describe an observable action, behavior, or achievement;

Measurable – there are systems, methods, or procedures to track or record the action upon which the objective is focused;

Achievable – the objective is realistic, based on current environment and resources;

Relevant – the objective is important to the program and is under the control of the program;

Time-based – there are clearly defined deadlines for achieving the objective.

The most recent and notable set of oral health objectives for the nation is included in the voluminous collection known as "Healthy People 2010 Objectives" [23], the third set of decennial United States health objectives. The chapter on oral health provides specific, measurable objectives to be achieved by the year 2010 to attain its stated goal: "Prevent and control oral and craniofacial diseases, conditions, and injuries and improve access to related services." Each oral health objective has a specified target population, a quantifiable measure to be attained, and a deadline. For example, the first objective is: "Reduce the proportion of young children with dental caries experience in their primary teeth. Target: 11 percent. Baseline: 18 percent of children aged 2 to 4 years had dental caries experience in 1988–94." Similarly, many states have established their own oral health objectives.

Once priorities have been established by the community oral health coalition and program goals and objectives have been agreed upon, the next step is to design and implement the program.

Implement the program

As with all previous steps, implementing a community oral health program requires the collaboration of individuals, organizations, and the community. Implementation involves identifying a series of specific activities that must occur to achieve the agreed-upon goals and objectives. Perhaps the most effective approach is to start with each objective and identify the activities that will be required to reach that objective. For example, one program objective might be: "By 2010, at least 50% of African-American men aged 35 years or older in Duval County, Florida, will report having been examined for oral cancer within the preceding 12 months." Achieving that objective would likely require several program components, as shown in the example in Table 1.

Each component of the program requires action steps to achieve that component's main outcome. Table 2 provides an example. One major advantage of establishing a community coalition to plan oral health programs

Table 1
Example of program components to achieve objective: "By 2010, at least 50% of African American men aged 35 years or older in Duval County will report having been examined for oral cancer within the preceding 12 months"

Program component	Target population	Desired outcome
Oral cancer awareness	African-American men aged ≥ 35 years	Increased knowledge of oral cancer risk factors, signs, symptoms
Accessibility of oral cancer examinations	African-American men aged ≥ 35 years	Attendance at oral cancer screenings
Quality of oral cancer examinations	Local dentists and dental hygienists	Increased competence in providing head and neck examinations

This objective was part of a community-based social marketing project designed to increase awareness of oral cancer, promote its earlier detection, and reduce racial disparities in stage at diagnosis and survival.

Data from Noland Dodd VJ, Watson JM, Choi Y, et al. Social marketing approach to increasing oral cancer exams among African-Americans [abstract 1266]. J Dent Res 2007;86:(Spec Iss A).

Table 2
Example of action steps needed to implement a program component in a community-based social marketing project designed to increase awareness of oral cancer, promote its earlier detection, and reduce racial disparities in stage at diagnosis and survival

Program component	Action step	Responsible entity	Target date
Oral cancer awareness	Determine target population and comparison community	County health department	February 1
	Conduct baseline survey in target and comparison communities	Survey research center	March 30
	Conduct formative focus groups in target population	Health education faculty at College of Public Health	April 30
	Design and test draft messages and materials	Faculty at College of Public Health and College of Dentistry	May 30
	Identify media and venues for dissemination	Community members of coalition	June 15
	Produce electronic and print materials	Health department communication office in collaboration with advertising agency	July 30
	Disseminate materials	Community organizations, professional organizations, county health department	August–November
	First follow-up survey in target and comparison communities	Survey research center	December 15

Data from Noland Dodd VJ, Watson JM, Choi Y, et al. Social marketing approach to increasing oral cancer exams among African-Americans [abstract 1266]. J Dent Res 2007;86:(Spec Iss A).

is that there are multiple individuals and organizations to help share in the implementation. If each entity assumes responsibility for one or a few activities, thereby sharing the burden, the program is more feasible than if one party with limited resources had to conduct all activities on its own.

Evaluate the program

It is essential that programs ensure that they are achieving the intended results, which requires program evaluation. Evaluation may be defined as systematic investigation of the merit, worth, or significance of an object [24,25]. Although Fig. 1 depicts program evaluation as one discrete step in the planning cycle, evaluation is an ongoing process that starts at program inception. Unfortunately, too many oral health programs are not adequately evaluated [26].

The ultimate purpose of the evaluation is to determine whether the program did what it was designed to do. There are, however, many other facets to consider. One classical framework for program evaluation, formulated by Donabedian [27], partitions the evaluation components into the broad categories of structure, process, and outcome. This framework has been employed in evaluations of community oral health programs [28,29]. *Structure* includes the physical aspects of the program, including facilities, equipment, personnel, finances, and logistics. *Process* includes the methods or techniques used to deliver the services. *Outcome* includes the impacts, effects, and changes that come about as a result of the program. Ideally, evaluations should include measures in all three components of the framework.

The CDC developed a practical framework for evaluating public health programs that encourages integrating evaluation with routine program operations [30]. The CDC framework takes into account three interrelated issues reflecting public health values: merit (ie, quality), worth (ie, cost-effectiveness), and significance (ie, importance). Even if a program is judged to be of merit, there may be questions as to whether the program is worth its cost. Also, there may be questions about whether even valuable programs are making significant differences.

The CDC framework has six steps that should be taken in any evaluation (Fig. 3) and are applied here to community oral health programs:

Step 1: Engage stakeholders

As described earlier regarding program development, effective community oral health work involves partnerships. Any evaluation of a community oral health program requires engaging the people and organizations that have an investment in the program, and clarifying what will be learned from the evaluation and what will be done with that information. After becoming involved, stakeholders help to carry out the other steps of the evaluation. The stakeholders include those involved in program operations (eg, sponsors, oral health coalition partners, managers, and staff); those served

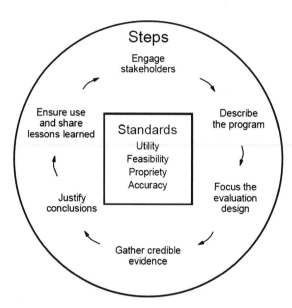

Fig. 3. CDC framework for program evaluation.

or affected by the program (eg, dental patients, neighborhood organizations, and local dentistry and dental hygiene associations); and the primary users of the evaluation (ie, the people who are in a position to do or decide something regarding the program).

Step 2: Describe the program

Program descriptions convey the mission and objectives of the program being evaluated. Descriptions should be sufficiently detailed to ensure understanding of program goals and strategies. The description should discuss the program's capacity to effect change, its stage of development (ie, a new initiative or a mature program), and how it fits into the larger organization and community. Program descriptions set the frame of reference for all subsequent decisions in an evaluation.

Step 3: Focus the evaluation design

The evaluation must be focused to assess the issues of greatest concern to stakeholders while using time and resources as efficiently as possible. Among the items to consider when focusing an evaluation are *purpose, users, uses, questions, methods,* and *agreements.*

Public health evaluations have four general *purposes*: (1) to gain insight from an innovative oral health program or practice; (2) to change practice, which is appropriate when an established community oral health program seeks to improve the quality, effectiveness, or efficiency of its activities; (3) to assess effects, by examining the relationship between program activities and outcomes; and (4) to affect those who participate in the inquiry by stimulating reflection of stakeholders and serving as a catalyst for self-directed change.

Users are the specific persons who will receive evaluation findings. User involvement is required for clarifying intended uses, prioritizing questions and methods, and preventing the evaluation from becoming misguided or irrelevant.

Uses are the specific ways in which information generated from the evaluation will be applied. Uses should be planned and prioritized with input from stakeholders, and all uses must be linked to one or more specific users.

Creating evaluation *questions* encourages the stakeholders to reveal what they believe the evaluation should answer. Negotiating and prioritizing questions among stakeholders further refines the focus of the evaluation.

The *methods* for an evaluation are drawn from scientific research options, and may include experimental, quasi-experimental, and observational study designs. The most appropriate design will largely depend on the question being asked, the feasibility of implementing the design, and acceptability to the users. No design is better than others under all circumstances. However, the choice of study design does have implications for the level of evidence that will be produced and the degree to which the findings will be generalizable. It is often desirable to include more than one study design in evaluating an oral health program.

Agreements clarify roles and responsibilities among those who will carry out the evaluation plan, and describe how the evaluation plan will be implemented by using available resources. Agreements also identify safeguards in place to protect human subjects and, where appropriate, ethical (eg, institutional review board) or administrative approvals.

Step 4: Gather credible evidence

An evaluation should strive to collect information that will present a well-rounded picture of the community oral health program so that the information is seen as credible by the evaluation's primary users. The evidence should be perceived by stakeholders as believable and relevant for answering their questions. Encouraging participation by stakeholders can also enhance perceived credibility. When stakeholders are involved in defining and gathering data that they find credible, they will be more likely to accept the evaluation's conclusions and to act on its recommendations [31,32]. Some of the aspects of evidence that may affect its perceived credibility include indicators, sources, quality, quantity, and logistics.

Indicators address criteria that will be used to judge the oral health program, and therefore should reflect aspects of the program that are meaningful to monitor. Examples of indicators that can be defined and tracked include measures of program activities (eg, participation rates, levels of patient satisfaction, the efficiency of resource use, and the amount of intervention exposure) and measures of program effects (eg, changes in participant behavior, community norms, policies or practices, health status, quality of life, and the settings or environment of the program).

Sources of evidence in an evaluation are the people, documents, or observations that provide information for the inquiry. Using multiple sources helps to include different perspectives about the program and will likely enhance the evaluation's credibility. Integrating qualitative and quantitative information can increase the chances that the evidence base will be balanced.

Quality refers to the appropriateness and integrity of the information used in an evaluation. High-quality data are reliable, valid, and informative for their intended use. Collecting quality data will involve consideration of factors such as study design, training of dental examiners or interviewers, and data cleaning and management.

Quantity refers to the amount of evidence gathered in an evaluation, which affects the potential confidence level or precision of the evaluation's conclusions. Determining the quantity of information to be collected often involves a balance among ensuring reasonable power to detect program effects, the burden placed on respondents, and the resources required to collect the data.

Logistics includes the methods, timing, and physical infrastructure for collecting and managing evidence. People and organizations may have cultural preferences that dictate acceptable ways of asking questions and collecting information, including who would be perceived as an appropriate person to ask the questions.

Step 5: Justify conclusions

The conclusions from a program evaluation are justified when they are linked to the evidence gathered and judged against agreed-upon values or standards set by the stakeholders. Justifying conclusions on the basis of evidence includes consideration of the stakeholders' values; analysis and synthesis of evidence from all sources; interpretation of those analyses; judgments on the merit, worth, and significance of the program; and development of recommendations for action, based on the evidence, that anticipate cultural and political sensitivities.

Step 6: Ensure use and share lessons learned

Lessons learned in the course of a program evaluation require specific efforts to ensure that the evaluation processes and findings are used and disseminated appropriately. Five elements are critical for ensuring use of an evaluation including design, preparation, feedback, follow-up, and dissemination. *Design* refers to how the evaluation's questions, methods, and overall processes are constructed, and should be organized from the start to achieve intended uses by primary users. *Preparation* includes the steps taken to rehearse eventual use of the evaluation findings, which could involve asking stakeholders to describe the actions they would take if they received a hypothetical set of results. *Feedback* is the communication that occurs among all stakeholders in the evaluation process. *Follow-up* involves providing technical and emotional support to assist users and remind them of the planned use of the evaluation's findings. *Dissemination* is the process of communicating the procedures or the lessons learned from an evaluation to relevant audiences in a timely, unbiased, and consistent manner.

Standards for effective evaluation

Finally, the CDC framework for evaluating public health programs identified 30 specific standards that should serve as guiding principles in designing an evaluation and guiding decisions among options [30]. These standards were grouped into four categories: utility, feasibility, propriety, and accuracy. *Utility standards* ensure that the evaluation will meet the information needs of the intended users. *Feasibility standards* ensure that an evaluation will be practical, politically viable, and cost-effective. *Propriety standards* ensure that an evaluation will be conducted legally, ethically, and with regard for the welfare of those involved in the evaluation as well as those affected by its results. Finally, *accuracy standards* ensure that an evaluation will produce findings that are considered technically correct.

Summary

Community oral health programs focus primarily on populations, including those who do not seek oral health care. Planning these programs should include involvement of the community, broadly defined to include individuals and organizations that represent those who can help design and implement it and those who could be affected by it. A systematic approach toward planning community oral health programs is advocated and includes identifying community oral health needs, assessing the available resources, determining the community's oral health priorities, setting measurable and achievable goals and objectives, implementing the program, and systematically evaluating the program. This approach helps to ensure that all stakeholders are in agreement on the purpose of the program, contribute toward its success, and provide constructive input toward its continuous improvement.

References

[1] American Academy of Pediatric Dentistry. Policy on the Dental Home. In: American Academy of Pediatric Dentistry Reference Manual 2005–2006. Chicago: American Academy of Pediatric Dentistry; 2006. p. 18–9.

[2] Jones K, Tomar SL. Estimated impact of competing policy recommendations for age of first dental visit. Pediatrics 2005;115(4):906–14.

[3] Stead LF, Lancaster T. Group behaviour therapy programmes for smoking cessation. Cochrane Database Syst Rev 2005;(2):CD001007.

[4] Burns DM. Smoking cessation: recent indicators of what's working at a population level. In: National Cancer Institute, editor. Population Based Smoking Cessation: Proceedings

of a Conference on What Works to Influence Cessation in the General Population. Smoking and Tobacco Monograph No. 12. NIH Publication No. 00-4892. Bethesda, MD: U.S. Department of Health and Human Services, National Institutes of Health, National Cancer Institute; 2000. p. 1–24.

[5] Truman BI, Gooch BF, Sulemana I, et al. Reviews of evidence on interventions to prevent dental caries, oral and pharyngeal cancers, and sports-related craniofacial injuries. Am J Prev Med 2002;23(Suppl 1):21–54.

[6] Marinho VCC, Higgins JPT, Logan S, et al. Fluoride varnishes for preventing dental caries in children and adolescents. Cochrane Database Syst Rev 2002;(Issue 1): Art. No.: CD002279. DOI: 10.1002/14651858:CD002279.

[7] Jones MM, Bayer R. Paternalism and its discontents: motorcycle helmet laws, libertarian values, and public health. Am J Public Health 2007;97(2):208–17.

[8] Baker SP. On lobbies, liberty, and the public good. Am J Public Health 1980;70(6):573–5.

[9] Martin B. Scientific knowledge in controversy: the social dynamics of the fluoridation debate. Albany (NY): State University of New York Press; 1991.

[10] Tickle M, Milsom KM, Buchanan K, et al. Dental screening in schools: the views of parents, teachers and school nurses. Br Dent J 2006;201(12):769–73 [discussion: 767].

[11] Mann ML. Planning for community dental programs. In: Gluck GM, Morganstein WM, editors. Jong's community dental health. 5th edition. St. Louis (MO): Mosby; 2003. p. 329–49.

[12] American Association for Community Dental Programs. A guide for developing and enhancing community oral health programs. Cincinnati (OH): American Association for Community Dental Programs; 2006.

[13] Washington State Department of Health. Community roots for oral health: guidelines for successful coalitions. Olympia (WA): Washington State Department of Health, Office of Maternal and Child Health, Oral Health Program; 2000.

[14] Institute of Medicine. Board of Health Promotion and Disease Prevention, Committee on Assuring the Health of the Public in the 21st Century. The future of the public's health in the 21st century. Washington, DC: National Academy Press; 2002.

[15] U.S. Census Bureau. American Community Survey [website]. Washington, D.C.: U.S. Census Bureau, American Community Survey Office; 2007. Available at: http://www.census.gov/acs/www/index.html. Accessed November 12, 2007.

[16] Association of State and Territorial Dental Directors. State & territorial dental public health activities: a collection of descriptive summaries. Acquiring oral health data [Web page]; 2007. Available at: http://www.astdd.org/index.php?template=sactnav_temp.php&;topic=Acquiring%20Oral%20Health%20Data Accessed June 1, 2007.

[17] Association of State and Territorial Dental Directors. Basic screening surveys: an approach to monitoring community oral health. Columbus (OH): Association of State and Territorial Dental Directors; 2003.

[18] Centers for Disease Control and Prevention. Health risks in the United States: Behavioral Risk Factor Surveillance System, 2007. Atlanta (GA): U.S. Department of Health and Human Services, Centers for Disease Control and Prevention, Coordinating Center for Health Promotion; 2007.

[19] Centers for Medicaid & Medicare Services. Federally qualified health center fact sheet. Washington, D.C.: U.S. Department of Health and Human Services, Centers for Medicaid & Medicare Services; 2007. Available at: http://www.cms.hhs.gov/MLNProducts/downloads/fqhcfactsheet.pdf. Accessed November 12, 2007.

[20] Health Resources and Services Administration. The Health Center Program: 2006 National Aggregate Uniform Data System Data. Table 2: Services Offered and Delivery Method. U.S. Department of Health and Human Services, Health Resources and Services Administration, Bureau of Primary Health Care; 2007. Available at: http://bphc.hrsa.gov/uds/2006data/national/nationaltable2.htm. Accessed November 12, 2007.

[21] National AHEC Organization. Area Health Education Centers/Health Education Training Centers: Connecting Students to Careers, Professionals to Communities, and Communities

to Better Health. Wexford (PA): National AHEC Organization; 2006. Available at: http://www.nationalahec.org/Publications/documents/2006%20NAO%20Brochure%2011x17.pdf. Accessed November 12, 2007.

[22] Drucker PF. The practice of management. New York: Harper; 1954.

[23] U.S. Department of Health and Human Services. Healthy People 2010. 2nd edition. With understanding and improving health and objectives for improving health, vol. 2. Washington, D.C.: U.S. Government Printing Office; 2000. Available at: http://www.healthypeople.gov/. Accessed November 12, 2007.

[24] Scriven M. Minimalist theory of evaluation: the least theory that practice requires. American Journal of Evaluation 1998;19(1):57–70.

[25] Shadish WR, Cook TD, Leviton LC. Foundations of program evaluation: theories of practice. Newbury Park (CA): Sage Publications; 1991.

[26] Watt R, Fuller S, Harnett R, et al. Oral health promotion evaluation–time for development. Community Dent Oral Epidemiol 2001;29(3):161–6.

[27] Donabedian A. The quality of care. How can it be assessed? JAMA 1988;260(12):1743–8.

[28] Hyde S, Weintraub JA, Satariano WA. An evaluation of the San Francisco department of human services welfare dental program. J Public Health Dent 2005;65(2):104–9.

[29] Vachirarojpisan T, Shinada K, Kawaguchi Y. The process and outcome of a programme for preventing early childhood caries in Thailand. Community Dent Health 2005;22(4):253–9.

[30] Centers for Disease Control and Prevention. Framework for program evaluation in public health. MMWR Recomm Rep 1999;48(RR-11):1–40.

[31] Patton MQ. Utilization-focused evaluation: the new century text. 3rd edition. Thousand Oaks (CA): Sage Publications; 1997.

[32] Fetterman DM, Kaftarian SJ, Wandersman A, editors. Empowerment evaluation: knowledge and tools for self-assessment and accountability. Thousand Oaks (CA): Sage Publications; 1996.

ELSEVIER
SAUNDERS

THE DENTAL
CLINICS
OF NORTH AMERICA

Dent Clin N Am 52 (2008) 423–446

Public Health Issues in Geriatric Dentistry in the United States

J.M. Chalmers, BDSc, MS, PhD*, R.L. Ettinger, BDS, MDS, DDSc

*Department of Preventive and Community Dentistry, College of Dentistry,
The University of Iowa, 810 Newton Road, Iowa City, IA 52242, USA*

Demographics of the aging population and epidemiology of their oral health

In the twentieth century, dramatic changes occurred with regard to health and disease, longevity, and mortality in the United States population. We have become an aging society. In 1900, 4% (3.1 million persons) of the United States population was aged 65 years or older and by 2005 it had increased to 34.3 million persons or 12.4% of the population, a more than tenfold increase [1]. The fastest growing sector of older adults is of those 80 years or older. Heterogeneity among persons 65 years of age or older is probably greater than at any other time period in the life span [2,3]. The challenges of life make older adults different from each other; yet all too often people aged 65 and older are considered as one homogeneous group when programs are planned.

Older adults are a complex combination and expression of their individual genetic predispositions, lifestyles, socialization, and environments; these factors affect health beliefs and impact health behavior. To treat an older adult, dentists must understand the cultural, psychologic, educational, social, economic, dietary, and chronologically related experiences that may have influenced that older person's life. Oral health is influenced by similar factors and is the accumulation of an individual's life experiences with dental care, as well as with caries, periodontal disease, and iatrogenic disease. Oral status reflects a history of the older person's behavioral attitudes and expectations for their own oral health. The skills, attitudes, and philosophies of the various dentists that persons may have encountered in their life spans will also affect oral status [4]. The oral health care of any of these older adults is termed "geriatric dentistry" and includes—but is not limited

* Corresponding author.
E-mail address: jane-chalmers@uiowa.edu (J.M. Chalmers).

0011-8532/08/$ - see front matter. Published by Elsevier Inc.
doi:10.1016/j.cden.2007.12.004

to—the diagnosis, treatment, and prevention of caries and periodontal disease, as well as oral mucosal diseases, head and neck pain, salivary dysfunction, and impaired chewing, tasting, and swallowing [5].

Older adults in the past comprised a relatively small proportion of the population; the majority of these people were edentulous and used dental care infrequently, and then only when previous unmet needs could no longer be ignored [6,7]. However, there is now adequate evidence to show that a new, older dental consumer has emerged, who is better educated, more politically aware and, more importantly, has some remaining natural teeth. Thus, the aging United States population living in the new millennium has dental needs that are very different and more complex than those experienced by previous older adult cohorts during the twentieth century. It is no longer appropriate to equate geriatric dental care with denture care, because care now must include complex restorative procedures as well as esthetic dentistry and implants [5,7].

For those older adults who are edentulous, oral health impacts are reported to be more frequent and affect chewing and food choice: they require ongoing dental care even when wearing complete dentures [8]. In the past 35 years the overall prevalence of edentulism in the United States has declined from 20.3% in 1972 to 13.9% in 2001 [9]. The most recent national data reported that 31.3% of people aged more than or equal to 75 years were edentulous, whereas the younger elderly (aged 65–74 years) have a prevalence of edentulism of 23.9% (Fig. 1) [10,11]. Edentulism also varies by state in the United States, with the highest prevalence of edentulism in 65 years or older adults in Kentucky (42.3%), West Virginia (41.9%), Tennessee (36%), and Mississippi (35.1%) [12]. The lowest prevalence of edentulism was

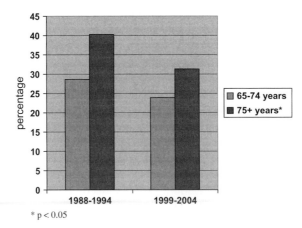

* $p < 0.05$

Fig. 1. Prevalence of edentulism among dentate seniors 65 or more years, United States, National Health and Nutrition Examination Survey (NHANES) 1988–1994 and 1999–2004. (*Data from* Dye BA, Tan S, Smith V, et al. Trends in oral health status: United States, 1988–1994 and 1999–2004. National Center for Health Statistics. Vital Health Stat 11 2007;(248).)

reported in Hawaii (13.1%), California (13.3%), Utah (14.7%), and Minnesota (14.8%) [12]. Retention of teeth is significantly higher in older adults with higher income and education levels, Hispanics and Whites, non-smokers, and those reporting excellent general health status [12]. A 2000 report indicated that tooth loss was highest in the United States among older American Indians and Alaskan Natives [13].

Older adults have been defined as a cohort of people aged 65 years or older. However, a chronologic definition of the aging population is not particularly useful in dentistry. A functional definition, based upon an older individual's ability to travel to seek services, is more appropriate; such a definition is also dynamic, with older adults often moving among the various categories as their health declines or improves [14]. The aging population can be functionally categorized into three broad groups: the functionally independent older adult, the frail older adult, and the functionally dependent older adult [15].

The majority of older adults (95%) live in the community; of these it can be estimated that around 5% are homebound and another approximately 17% have a major limitation in mobility because of some chronic condition. This still leaves about 73% of the population over the age of 65 years who are living in the community and are able to come to the dental office independently [6,14]. Approximately 5% are institutionalized; over 1.65 million older Americans reside in nursing homes [6,14]. Nearly half of nursing home residents are aged 85 or more years [6,14]. These residents have high levels of functional dependence combined with high levels of cognitive impairment. Assistance with three or more activities of daily living is needed by more than 75% of residents, such as showering or bathing (including oral hygiene care), dressing, and eating. Cognitive impairment is evident in more than 70% of residents [16].

Coronal and root caries

National data detailing the oral health status of older Americans reveal some interesting trends over time. Mean number of permanent teeth among dentate older adults aged 65 or more years have increased between the National Health and Nutrition Examination Survey (NHANES) round III (1988–1994) and that conducted in 1999 to 2004, especially in the aged 75 or more cohort, and those with higher incomes, better education, and non-smokers (Fig. 2). Mean number of decayed, missing, and filled teeth in older Americans aged 65 or more years have decreased slightly across these surveys, including the contribution of decayed coronal surfaces [10]. NHANES comparison data from rounds I (1971–1974) and III (1988–1994) reported that the percentage of teeth with caries (treated or untreated) decreased for participants aged 18 to 54 years but increased for participants aged 55 to 74 years [17]. The overall prevalence of coronal caries in older adults aged 65 or more years did not significantly change between NHANES

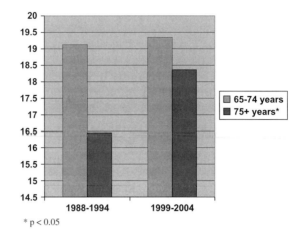

Fig. 2. Mean number of permanent teeth among dentate seniors aged 65 or more years, United States, NHANES 1988–1994 and 1999–2004. (*Data from* Dye BA, Tan S, Smith V, et al. Trends in oral health status: United States, 1988–1994 and 1999–2004. National Center for Health Statistics. Vital Health Stat 11 2007;(248).)

rounds in 1988 to 1994 and 1999 to 2004, but the prevalence of untreated dental caries overall in older Americans significantly decreased, with higher untreated caries prevalence evident in older African Americans and Hispanics, those with lower incomes, less education, and current or former smokers. This was also the case for untreated root caries [10]. Greater retention of teeth predisposes many older adults to a continual risk of both new and recurrent coronal and root caries, and extends the risk for developing gingivitis and periodontal diseases [18]. Dental caries is still clearly a public health problem for subgroups of older Americans, such as those of lower socioeconomic status, with dementia, who are homebound and who are institutionalized [14,19,20].

Periodontal and oral mucosal diseases

Removal of dental plaque becomes a more difficult challenge because of age-related toothbrush abrasion, gingival recession, salivary dysfunction, dexterity disabilities, and cognitive impairment [18]. The prevalence and incidence of periodontal conditions in older adults has clearly been related to poor oral hygiene and high levels of dental plaque [8]. Data from the NHANES surveys has reported a significant increase in mean recession in older adults, but a significant decrease in mean pocket depth and mean loss of attachment, and in severe periodontal disease (Fig. 3). Mean loss of attachment was significantly higher in older males, older African and Hispanic Americans, in poorer older Americans, those older adults with less than high school education, and older current or former smokers [10]. A variety of oral mucosal conditions may be present in older adults, and may be

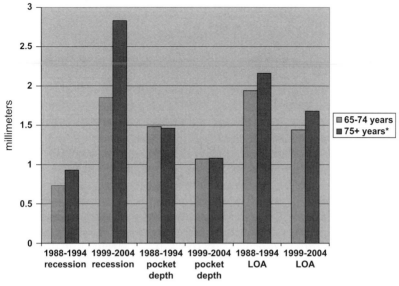

* p < 0.05 between 1988-1994 and 1999-2004

Fig. 3. Mean recession, pocket depth and loss of attachment among dentate seniors aged 65 or more years, United States, NHANES 1988–1994 and 1999–2004. (*Data from* Dye BA, Tan S, Smith V, et al. Trends in oral health status: United States, 1988–1994 and 1999–2004. National Center for Health Statistics. Vital Health Stat 11 2007;(248).)

exacerbated by salivary dysfunction. Oral and pharyngeal cancer in particular are relevant to older Americans, with the median age at diagnosis at 64 years; the primary determinants of this cancer are smoking and alcohol use [17].

Geriatric access, barriers, and use of dental care in the United States: models of care provision

The aging United States population is a "looming and major challenge that will exacerbate the issue of access to care" in dentistry [21]. Older adults are seeking dental care at a growing rate. Locker [22] and others have evidenced that "improvements in the oral health of older adults depend upon access to comprehensive dental treatments." Indeed, the type of dental care needing to be provided for older adults goes way beyond emergency care and denture care, as was discussed by Barmes [23]: "...public policies to support community awareness and acceptance of broad-based preventive behaviors to preserve oral health in old age are essential. Policies also must provide guidance on how to... ensure access to cost-effective and high-quality services for all."

The percentage of community-living older Americans who visited the dentist within the past year is steadily increasing and is expected to continue to do so for several decades. However, a lower percentage of older adults

(56.3% in 2004) visited the dentist within the past year, in comparison to adults (64.0% in 2004) and children (76.4%). The lowest use was reported for the poorest older adults and for older African Americans. Data also indicated that rural older Americans were less likely to report being regular dental care users than urban older Americans. Data from the 2006 United States National Health Interview Survey indicated that 71.69% of dentate persons 75 years and older had been to the dentist within the last year. However, only 17.8% of edentulous adults over age 65 had such a visit [24]. The majority (59.2%) of these edentulous older adults had not used the services of a dentist for at least 5 years. Older adults with some natural teeth were using dental services in a manner similar to younger adults. The value older adults place on dental care seems to influence use more than any other factor, including their ability to pay for care [25]. Data from the 1996 Medical Expenditure Survey confirmed that persons over age 65 used more restorative, prosthetic, and oral surgery services than any other age group [26]. Another study examined dental service use by independent living adults in private practice, and showed that older adults sought dental services at rates greater than those expected by their representative percentage [27]. It was also reported that "patient visits by older adults generated, on average, as much or more income than did visits by individuals from any other age grouping" [28].

Several other barriers to dental care for older Americans include lack of perceived need, poor health literacy, and inadequate federal policies and regulations. There is a clearly reduced perceived need for dental care and dental use by edentulous older adults versus dentate older adults. Perceived need is also reduced as functional dependency increases, and dental care use concurrently decreases, especially in those older adults who are institutionalized [14,29]. Some reviews have highlighted reduced perceived need as the greatest barrier to dental care use in older adult cohorts [29]. Another less studied barrier is that of poor health literacy; this is reflected in challenges for older adults with accessing dental services, performing oral hygiene tasks, completing fully informed consent procedures, participating actively in decision-making in dental treatment planning, and undertaking follow-up oral health care activities [30]. Despite the enactment of federal legislation in 1987 mandating that nursing homes provide access to dental care for residents, the poor oral health status and use data reported in recent years evidenced that adequate access to dental care does not exist for many United States nursing home residents [14]. Thus, the treatment older adults seek will depend directly upon their self-perceived need, their financial ability to pay for that care, and issues such as transportation and documentation, rather than the normative need detected during an oral examination by a dentist [29,31].

The Agency for Health care Research and Quality reported in 2000 that older adults aged 65 or more years paid 75% or more of their dental expenses out-of-pocket, compared with the general population out-of-pocket expenses of around 50% [32]. The main reason for this large out-of-pocket expense in older Americans is the lack of reimbursement for dental care; after retirement, dental insurance is often only available for older adults with retiree plans, which is a minority of the older population [14,33,34]. Routine dental care is generally not covered by Medicare, and Medicaid coverage varies greatly between states [14,33,34].

In an analysis of the Asset of Health Dynamics Among the Oldest Old dataset from 1993 to 1995, it was clear that economic access factors had a strong indirect effect on dental use disparities among African Americans and Hispanics, because of the fact that dental services were not covered by Medicare [29,35]. This analysis indicated that Medicare played a very important role in providing older minority Americans with access to medical care, and the lack of Medicare dental coverage was a barrier to them accessing dental care [35]. One of the greatest barriers to care for Medicaid recipients is that the reimbursement rate is so low that many dentists are discouraged from treating Medicaid patients, especially those in nursing homes [14,16,36,37]. Rubinstein [34] portrays the current situation succinctly: "Americans are concerned about access to health care and the cost of prescription drugs, (but) Americans' interest in increased access to dental care for seniors never registers." A suggested solution is the increased use of tax-deferred dental or medical savings accounts, where balances accrue over time and then can be accessed later in life. Others have suggested a Medicare dental supplemental insurance program, with an emphasis on preventive dental services, or a dental insurance plan that is prepaid during employment similar to long-term care insurance [38,39].

Stakeholder partnerships to improve access to dental care

There will be many challenges in reducing barriers and improving access to and use of dental care for older Americans in the coming years. Stakeholders, including dental professionals and the dental benefits industry, need to develop innovative dental financing programs that will increase older Americans access to dental care. Most dental services for older adults are provided in community-based offices by private dental practitioners. For functionally independent and frail older adults, a few modifications in office design to allow for normal aging changes will allow private practitioners to treat this population [40]. For nonambulatory dependent older adults, including nursing home residents, a variety of dental service delivery system models are needed, which involve several stakeholder partnerships.

The most common model used to provide dental care for dependent older adults is transporting them to a dental office, which is the most convenient for dental professionals as they can treat patients in their own offices with auxiliary personnel and appropriate equipment [37]. It is also the most cost-effective service for a dentist, as no traveling or set-up time is required, but it is expensive and time-consuming for a nursing home, as a staff member needs to accompany their resident to the dental office. Thus, not surprisingly, many nursing homes are reluctant to contract such an arrangement, and thus little care under these circumstances is voluntarily offered to nursing home residents. Transporting dependent older adults requires a suitable vehicle and use of volunteer drivers, subsidized transport, or ambulances, which creates many coordination, organization, and financing problems for both the patient and nursing home. Many modifying factors need to be considered when transporting a dependent older adult to a dentist's office: the person's activity level, continence, transferability appointment times, accompanying person, communication, legal consent issues, and ethical considerations.

There are some excellent partnerships that have been formed on regional levels across the United States, between private dental practitioners and local nursing homes, in which the nursing home provides a "dental office" with a dental chair and other required dental equipment. The equipment may be owned by the nursing home or the dentist, or may have been donated. The main advantage of this partnership model is that residents can be treated within their own environment, for it has been shown that frail and cognitively impaired older adults do not withstand well the disruption of being transported, and disruptive behaviors often result when they are taken out of their nursing home setting. Some disadvantages are that the "fixed" dental equipment may not be able to be used bedside, and that the nursing home needs to be large (150 or more residents) to ensure financial success of the dental program. A modification of this model is when the dental professional brings portable dental equipment with them each visit, but the nursing home has a fixed dental chair that is also used for other purposes, such as for aromatherapy or podiatry. Several comprehensive reviews of portable and mobile dental equipment have been published [41–43].

A very successful partnership model in the United States has been that of larger groups of dental practitioners working together as a not-for-profit entity, using a combination of portable and mobile dental equipment. Longstanding examples of this model are Apple Tree Dental in Minnesota (http://www.appletreedental.org), and Access Dental and Carolina's Mobile Dentistry in North Carolina (http://www.accessdentalcare.org/http://www.carolinas.org/services/seniorcare/mobileDentistry.cfm). Another variation of this model is when the dental professionals include dental students from dental schools (some examples include the University of Iowa, Ohio State University, University of British Columbia, Marquette University, University of Southern California, and University of Minnesota).

Additional stakeholders in these programs have included state dental associations, state government public health and aging entities, and dental insurance companies. In these programs, dentists, dental hygienists, and dental assistants work together to provide dental treatment on-site at nursing homes and other sites for older adults. A variety of light and heavier portable equipment is transported in a truck or recreational vehicle from site to site. The program stays at a nursing home site for several weeks or months to provide comprehensive dental treatment for residents. A room is provided by the nursing home for the setting-up of the portable dental clinic, which includes dental chairs, portable high-speed dental units, portable headrests for wheelchairs, and portable x-ray equipment. These larger partnership models have gradually replaced mobile dental vans, which were often used in the 1970s and 1980s to provide dental treatment at nursing homes. The many disadvantages of the mobile vans included initial capital costs, weather conditions, and the electrical capacity of the motor home. Many residents are stressed when they are moved from the controlled environment of a facility through inclement weather into the mobile van.

One of the largest and nationally focused stakeholder partnerships in geriatric dentistry is that between GlaxoSmithKline Consumer Health care, the American Dental Association (ADA), and the ADA Foundation, which have entered into a 3-year $1 million national partnership to help address the oral health needs of aging Americans. These partners, together with the Special Care Dentistry Association, will present the upcoming OralLongevity series at the ADA national meeting in 2007, with an accompanying brochure and DVD education program for dental professionals to use with older adults and caregivers.

Interactions among state dental associations, state dental public health officials, academicians, and private practitioners have resulted in some productive partnerships to improve access to dental care for frail and dependent older adults. In these partnerships, links and communication have been established and maintained among dental professionals and nursing homes. Some also involving the sharing of portable dental equipment, as well as handbooks containing policies and procedures such as contracts, oral hygiene care manuals, and other reference materials (some examples are the Iowa Dental Association, British Columbia Dental Association, Louisville Dental Society, and North Carolina Dental Society with Carolina's Mobile Dentistry). Another example of such a stakeholder partnership is Iowa's Seniors Smiles project, coordinated by the Iowa Department of Public Health, Oral Health Bureau, and the University of Iowa, which links Medicaid waiver program homebound older adults and local dental professionals with the support of the home nursing program. In the Iowa program, oral health screenings by nurses identify homebound older adults with dental needs, and nurses are trained in preventive oral hygiene care activities to use with their older clients.

Geriatric oral health promotion

Geriatric oral health promotion in the new millennium

Traditionally, there has been very limited geriatric oral health promotion, with several myths contributing to this situation; the main focus has been on geriatric health education and assessment of normative dental needs [44]. Contemporary geriatric oral health promotion in the new millennium has an evidence-based and planned approach. As concluded by Watt and colleagues [45], "a standardized set of appropriate validated outcome measures is needed to assess the full impact of oral health promotion actions" using "both quantitative and qualitative methods." Contemporary geriatric oral health promotion encompasses not only the treatment of oral diseases and conditions, but has an increased focus on the prevention of oral diseases and conditions to enhance oral health status and older adults' quality of life. Various settings need to be used in addition to the traditional dental practice, including medical practices, people's homes, and residential care settings. Geriatric oral health promotion requires interdisciplinary involvement of medical, allied health, and dental professionals across these settings. Access to older adults is via community groups, support services, government organizations, families, and caregivers. Increased advocacy and involvement of these groups in regulatory and policy issues results in the strengthening of community action about geriatric oral health issues.

Functional geriatric oral health promotion matrix

Using the World Health Organization (WHO) Ottawa Charter/Jakarta Declaration and Ettinger's functional dependence classification, a geriatric oral health promotion matrix is presented (Table 1) [44]. The WHO Jakarta Declaration has identified that using combinations of the principles of the Ottawa Charter is more successful than their individual use. The five principles are to: (1) build health public policy; (2) create supportive environments; (3) strengthen community action; (4) develop personal skills; and (5) reorient health services. There are several activities that can be performed under each of these principles to provide a framework for oral health promotion and education interventions, with an evaluation component. For example, building healthy public policy involves advocacy from a large group of stakeholders from the community and health professions to improve financial access to dental care for older adults. Another example is to strengthen community action and develop the personal skills of health professionals to implement interdisciplinary oral health screenings for older adults. For functionally independent older adults this may be via regular check-ups with medical physicians, and for frail and dependent older adults this may be via regular interactions with nursing personnel.

Dental education models in geriatric dentistry and provision of care

Rational treatment planning

Maintaining adequate oral health is essential for older adults for their quality of life and for medical reasons. Older adults need to eat and talk comfortably, to feel happy with their appearance, to stay pain free, to maintain self-esteem, and to maintain habits and standards of hygiene and care that they have had throughout their life [46]. Behavioral problems, such as disinterest in food and not eating, "pulling" at the face or mouth, chewing of the lip, tongue or hands, grinding of teeth or dentures, not wearing of dentures, aggression (especially during activities of daily living), and alterations in activity (such as somnolence, tiring, screaming, and restlessness) can be caused by dental pain and problems. Adequate oral hygiene and dental treatment are needed to prevent medical problems, such as aspiration pneumonia and bacteremias; to manage medication side-effects, such as dry-mouth, speech problems, swallowing problems, tardive dyskinesia, and gingival overgrowth; to maintain adequate nutrition and hydration; and to manage consequences of comorbid medical conditions, such as Sjogren's syndrome, arthritis, strokes, radiation, and chemotherapy [46].

Rational dental treatment planning reviews all of the patient's modifying factors together with oral environmental factors, and to develop a realistic dental treatment plan for frail and dependent older adults. Such modifying factors include the patient's and their caregiver or family desires and expectations; the patient's medical or neurologic conditions and current or past medications; the patient's financial, social, transport, and residential situation; the patient's ability to tolerate the stress of treatment; the type and severity of the patient's dental pain and dental needs; how the dental problems affect the patient's quality of life; the patient's ability to maintain oral hygiene care; the probability of positive treatment outcomes; the availability of reasonable and less-extensive treatment alternatives; the dental team's ability to deliver the care needed (skills and equipment available); and other issues (for example, the patient's lifespan, bioethical issues) [47].

In the overall context of geriatric minimal intervention dentistry, consideration is also needed of a group of primary oral factors and plaque or biofilm factors before a final rational dental treatment plan is formulated (Fig. 4) [48]. A rational dental treatment plan may include several care options and is dynamic. It is important that introductory geriatric dentistry curricula incorporate case-based patient scenarios for training in rational dental treatment planning.

Undergraduate and graduate training models

There is a core of older American dentists who did not receive clinical or didactic training in geriatric dentistry, but who have provided some dental care for frail and dependent older patients. Most of this care has been provided at their dental offices, rather than off-site in patients' homes or in nursing homes [33,37]. In a recent interview study, these dentists emphasized the importance of providing "practical experience for learning how to manage patients with physical and/or cognitive disabilities" [33]. This interview study also highlighted that younger dentists have received some training

Table 1
Geriatric oral health promotion matrix for older adults

Principles of the Ottawa charter	Increasing functional dependency		
	Independent	Frail	Dependent
Build healthy public policy	Political advocacy to improve financial access to care (eg, retirees, Medicare)	Protocols and standards for home-based care	Protocols and enforcement of standards for facility-based care
	Recognition of specialty in geriatric dentistry	Improving government funded dental reimbursement for homebound (eg, Medicaid)	Improving government funded dental reimbursement for nursing homes (eg, Medicaid)
Create supportive environments	Fluoridation-specific geriatric dental health information (eg, liaisons with geriatric education centers)	Dental aids	Funding of geriatric dental services for institutionalized and hospitalized older adults
		Specific geriatric dental health information	Caregiver and agency education: curricula in oral health
		Funding of geriatric dental services for homebound older adults	

Strengthen community action	Directories of geriatric dental services Dissemination of oral health messages via community groups (eg, Alzheimers' Association; seniors centers)	Interdisciplinary oral health screening assessments in the community Linking homebound older adults with dental services via home nurses and other health professionals	Interdisciplinary oral health screening assessments in institutions Directories of geriatric dental services for nursing homes (eg, links with state dental associations)
Develop personal skills	Personalized oral hygiene skill development for older adults	Health professionals developing skills to implement oral health screenings for older patients; caregiver oral hygiene skill development Patient education in retaining oral hygiene care abilities	Health professionals developing skills to implement oral health screenings for older patients; caregiver oral hygiene skill development
Reorient health services	Geriatric minimal dental intervention Preventive oral health care	Geriatric minimal dental intervention Preventive oral health care Mobile and portable dental services: provision of care on-site at homes and facilities	Geriatric minimal dental intervention Geriatric atraumatic dental technique Preventive oral health care Mobile and portable dental services: provision of care on-site at homes and facilities

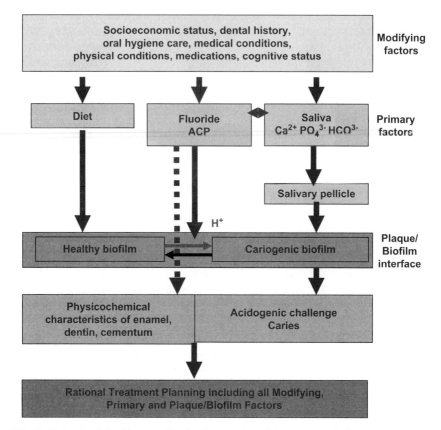

Fig. 4. Geriatric minimal intervention dentistry. (*Adapted from* Ngo H, Gaffney S. Risk assessment in the diagnosis and management of caries. In: Mount GJ, Hume WR, editors. Preservation and restoration of tooth structure. Brisbane, Australia: Knowledge Books and Software; 2005; with permission.)

in geriatric dentistry, but still many of them are not very interested in providing dental care off-site from their dental offices. A group of these younger dentists are using portable equipment to provide dental care on-site in nursing homes.

In a survey of all United States dental schools in 2003, it was reported that although 98% had didactic curricula in geriatric dentistry, only two-thirds had a specific undergraduate geriatric dentistry curriculum that included practical training and clinical rotation in the geriatric community. The content of the didactic component varied greatly. The clinical component was elective in 23% of these dental schools. Thirty percent reported having a specific geriatric dental clinic in the dental school and 11% had a remote clinical site. Most of the teaching in geriatric dentistry was shared among multiple departments. Two-thirds of dental schools had a geriatric program director or a chairman of a geriatric section [49]. Although increasing, there are insufficient curricula in geriatric dentistry in many dental hygiene training courses. As stated by Robbertz and colleagues [33], "providers need to be well-trained and confident in their ability to manage the older adult from both a psychologic and a clinical perspective." Educational research has substantiated this, highlighting that students' attitudes and knowledge toward older adults were not as important as their perceptions and confidence in providing dental care [50,51]. Examples of United States and Canadian dental schools with comprehensive geriatric dentistry didactic and clinical models include: The University of Iowa, Ohio State University, University of British Columbia, Marquette University, University of Southern California, University of Colorado, and the University of Minnesota. A comprehensive geriatric dentistry curriculum resource guide has been produced by the American Dental Education Association, with the support of Glaxo SmithKline Consumer Health care (http://www.adea.org/cepr/Documents/CurriculumResourceGuide.pdf).

Pyle and colleagues [36] concluded that for tomorrow's dental students to be prepared to face the challenges presented by aging population, "new (interdisciplinary) models of curricula in dentistry, medicine and allied health professions must emerge" that will consider the whole patient. This has been the premise underlying the development of the Health Resources and Services Administration interdisciplinary geriatric fellowship program Faculty Training Projects in Medicine, Dentistry, and Behavioral Medicine. This 1- or 2-year program trains geriatric medicine, psychiatry, and dentistry fellows together in the areas of administration, teaching, research, cultural competence, and clinical care. This program was halted in 2005 but then reinstated in 2007. There are not clear numbers available to determine the number of fellows trained in recent years, but the number is much reduced from the hundred or more fellows who were trained in Veterans Administration and other geriatric postgraduate programs in the late 1980s–early 1990s [36]. Another mechanism for some training in geriatric dentistry has been via hospital-based 1-year training programs for new graduates, but interest in these programs is waning [18].

According to Vargas and colleagues [52], "Optimally, the elderly should receive care from specialists in geriatric dentistry or general dentists with a good understanding of the medical, pharmacologic, and cognitive changes associated with the older population." However, geriatric dentistry is not currently one of the nine ADA recognized dental specialties in the United States. There are several other countries that have instituted specialty registration in geriatric and special needs dentistry (Australia, New Zealand, and Brazil), and progress has been made toward specialty recognition in the United Kingdom.

Evidence for therapeutic interventions for oral diseases in older adults

There are many clinical and restorative challenges for dentists treating older patients, including erosion, abrasion, demineralization, rampant coronal and root caries, retained roots, recurrent caries (crowns, repairs), subgingival caries, wet oral environments, saliva dysfunction, patient disruptive behaviors, poor compliance with preventive care, high plaque levels, and financial and other restrictions on care options [48]. To manage these challenges, many preventive and therapeutic dental interventions have been advocated, including fluoridated water, fluoride toothpastes (1,000 ppm and 5,000 ppm), fluoride gels, fluoride mouthrinses, antimicrobials (in mouthwash, gel, and varnish forms such as chlorhexidine gluconate, essential oils, cetylpyridinium chloride, decapinol), xylitol, amorphous calcium phosphates, and saliva substitutes or stimulants (see Fig. 4) [48,53]. However, published evidence for the use of these regimens for oral diseases in adults is generally limited in comparison with child populations. The greatest amount of evidence is available for caries prevention, with the use of fluoridated water (with an optimal fluoride concentration) and regular toothbrushing with a fluoridated 1,000 ppm dentrifice [54,55].

There is an increasing, but still small, amount of research being conducted with preventive and therapeutic regimens in older adults, especially dependent and behaviorally difficult older adults [56]. Neutral sodium fluoride products are used in older patients in preference to acidulated and stannous fluorides, mainly because of the adverse effects that the two latter products have on dental materials, such as composite and porcelain [48]. High fluoride containing toothpastes (5,000 ppm) have shown therapeutic effect on root caries in older adults [57]. Increasing evidence is supporting the regular use of fluoride varnish (26,000 ppm fluoride) for the management and prevention of dental caries, including in high-risk older adult populations [58,59]. However, there has been inadequate research conducted on root caries and recurrent caries in older populations in particular [56]. Some caries clinical trials have been conducted in older adults with chlorhexidine gluconate (CHX); the best results were achieved with the use of CHX varnish (10%) and gel (1%) rather than mouth rinse (0.12%) [60–62]. There is some evidence that the combined effect of CHX and fluoride varnish is even greater than either one used alone [60]. CHX trials have shown reduction in plaque accumulation and related indices, including the use of the 0.12% mouth rinse in a spray bottle for older adults. Frequency of CHX mouth rinse application has traditionally been twice daily; however, there is evidence that once daily is adequate [63]. Although there is increasing evidence for the caries therapeutic effect of amorphous calcium phosphate products, only one study to date has shown this effect in an adult population with salivary gland dysfunction [64,65].

Saliva substitutes and buffers are buffering, rehydrating, or mucosal protective products to help replace the functions and feeling of the missing saliva [66]. A range of substitutes are available as gels, liquids, and sprays from a variety of distributors. There are a few studies that evidence some improvement of xerostomia symptoms (self-perceived dry mouth), but these have been conducted mainly with radiation and cancer patients rather than specific older adult populations [67,68]. Saliva stimulant medications, such as pilocarpine and cevimeline, have improved saliva flow in clinical studies, but all have significant side effects (particularly on the cardiovascular system), and it is advisable to consult a patient's medical practitioner before prescribing such medications. Even preventive screening for oral cancer in older adults has not been yet evidenced to improve health outcomes, nor have the benefits and harms of such a screening been elucidated [56].

Models of geriatric homebound and nursing home dental care provision

Geriatric oral health triad

There is abundant international data to evidence that homebound and institutionalized older adults have the poorest oral health of nearly any group in society. The preservation of the natural dentition for these older adults requires three key components of a geriatric oral health triad be addressed: (1) regular oral assessment; (2) regular oral hygiene care; and (3) provision of dental treatment. MacEntee's research has highlighted the importance of a "dental champion" in the nursing home for the provision of successful dental treatment and oral hygiene care [69,70].

Role of the dental hygienist

A key participant in the delivery of geriatric oral health care is the dental hygienist. The hygienist performs any clinical hygiene procedure necessary (as is permitted by regional dental board regulations) and develops and maintains oral hygiene care plans for each resident. They provide hands-on regular inservice training and support for the nursing home staff, assist the staff to incorporate oral hygiene care into residents' personal care plans, and assist in the administration of dental policies and procedures [44,46]. The hygienist is central to the coordination of the nursing home dental program with the identified nursing home "dental champion." The hygienist works in an interdisciplinary team with medical, nursing, dietary, and other nursing home staff to ensure regular dental screening of residents. Gradually, more regions in the United States and other countries are introducing independent practice for dental hygienists in nursing homes, and regional regulations concerning this need to be obtained from administrative regional dental boards. There needs to be sufficient hygiene curricula and continuing education available to ensure adequate training in geriatric dentistry.

Role of the dentist of record

All United States nursing homes with federal funding are required to have a dentist of record who has a contractual agreement with them to carry out regular comprehensive dental examinations and emergency or comprehensive dental treatment for all of its consenting residents [71]. The dentist of record works with the administrator, the director of nursing, and the medical director or consultant to develop a dental program that suits the policy and procedural needs of the nursing home. A dental program policy agreement needs to incorporate the following points, while also incorporating regional regulations (eg, Minimum Data Set or similar guidelines or standards):

- All residents must have a dentist of record.
- Participation by competent residents in a dental program must be voluntary, but the institution should have an initial dental screening of all residents at or about the time of admission, which is documented in the resident's record and can be performed by a medical practitioner, a registered nurse, a hygienist, or a dentist.
- The initial short dental screening should be followed by a thorough dental examination by a dentist within 6 weeks of admission.
- Both dentate and edentulous residents should have a dental and oral examination at least once yearly.
- A written policy for oral hygiene care for its residents should be in place.

Caregivers—influences on their oral hygiene care provision

Residents' functional dependence and cognitive impairment results in their inability to regularly perform their own oral hygiene care, and thus their dependence on caregivers [16]. In nursing homes, these caregivers are generally certified nursing assistants (CNAs); licensed practical nurses (LPNs) and registered nurses (RNs) supervise them and RNs only provide oral hygiene care if it is a prescribed product (eg, 5,000 ppm fluoride toothpaste). Both CNAs and RNs have limited training and knowledge concerning oral diseases and oral hygiene care, especially care provision for residents with disruptive or care-resistant behaviors and communication problems [16,72]. Caregivers are scared of these behaviors and of being injured themselves or of inadvertently injuring the resident. Inadequate staff to resident ratios and insufficient time to complete tasks results in oral hygiene care often being neglected or falling to the bottom of the priority list [72,73]. Oral hygiene care is a less visible care task that cannot be easily evaluated and traced back to individual caregivers [74]. Recent United States research has revealed that even less oral hygiene care is likely being provided than has been previously reported [75].

Coleman and Watson [75], using a blinded observational study design, reported that very few CNAs wore gloves during oral hygiene care activities, and if they did wear gloves they were not changed inbetween various different care activities (eg, toileting, dressing, oral hygiene care, and so forth). CNAs are paid minimum wage and their job turnover is over 400% annually; many stay working in a nursing home for less than a year, although there is often a small core of CNAs that have worked for 5 to 10 years [76,77]. Many CNAs have poor oral health themselves, and may have experienced poor access to dental care. A model detailing these influences on poor oral hygiene care provision is presented in Fig. 5. In this model, four cycles (resident-medical, resident-dental, caregive-nursing home, and dental care) feed off one another to perpetuate poor oral hygiene care in nursing homes [73].

There have been many successful international inservice training programs for CNAs, which have evaluated both the short and long-term effectiveness of the program on residents' oral health [77–81]. The traditional single annual dental inservice has not been evidenced as successfully improving residents' oral health. A key component of the more successful programs has been hands-on training in small groups, by a dentist or dental hygienist, on a regular weekly or monthly basis [82]. Newer training programs developed for CNAs educational curricula have a story-based focus rather than the traditional "show and tell of bad mouths" [83]. CNAs require very basic skills in organization, preparation, and execution of activities, rather than intensive knowledge of oral diseases, to provide adequate oral hygiene care. LPNs and RNs require more knowledge of oral diseases. Key skills for caregivers are needed in communication and behavior management strategies for dementia [56,84]. Regular implementation of interdisciplinary screening oral assessments is needed by nondental nursing home staff and

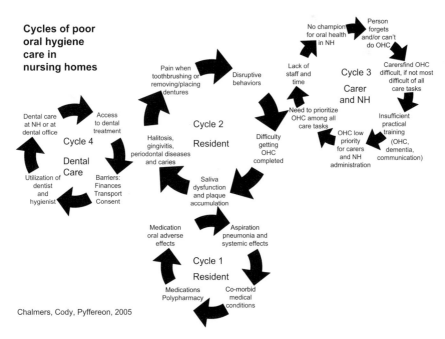

Fig. 5. Model of cycles of poor oral hygiene care in nursing homes. OHC, oral hygiene care. (*From* Pyfferoen M, Cody K, Chalmers J, et al. Observation of mealtime and oral hygiene cares for dementia residents. J Dent Res 2007;86(Spec Iss A):955. Available at: http://iadr.confex. com/iadr/2007orleans/techprogram/abstract_88327.htm; with permission.)

physicians. Several of these have been validated and can be individualized to suit regional policies and procedures [56,84,85]. It is essential that each screening assessment tool have an accompanying training program [84,86].

Summary

The aging United States population living in the new millennium has dental needs that are very different and more complex than those experienced by previous older adult cohorts during the twentieth century. The type of dental care to be provided for older Americans goes way beyond emergency care, extractions, and denture care. The prevalence and incidence of periodontal conditions in older adults has clearly been related to poor oral hygiene and high levels of dental plaque. Data from the NHANES surveys has reported a significant increase in mean recession in older adults, but a significant decrease in mean pocket depth and mean loss of attachment, and in severe periodontal disease.

Dental caries is still clearly a public health problem for subgroups of older Americans, such as those of lower socioeconomic status, with dementia, who are homebound and who are institutionalized. These are also the subgroups experiencing greater barriers to accessing dental care. The percentage of community-living older Americans who visited the dentist within the past year is steadily increasing and will continue to do so for several decades. Stakeholders, including dental professionals and the dental benefits industry need to work together to develop innovative dental financing programs that will increase older Americans' access to dental care. Most dental services for older adults are provided in community-based offices by private dentists. For nonambulatory, frail, and dependent older adults, a variety of dental service delivery system models are needed. Although 98% of United States dental schools in 2003 had didactic curricula in geriatric dentistry, only two-thirds had a specific undergraduate curriculum that included practical training and clinical rotation. There are a large number of preventive and therapeutic regimens advocated for use in treating oral diseases in older adults. However, published evidence for their use in older adults is limited. The preservation of the natural dentition for functionally dependent older adults requires three key components of a geriatric oral health triad be addressed: (1) regular oral assessment; (2) regular oral hygiene care; and (3) provision of dental treatment. Further research and intervention trials are needed concerning these three components in United States nursing homes.

References

[1] U.S. Census Bureau, Population Projections Branch. National Population Projections I Summary Files. Total Population by Age, Sex, Race, and Hispanic Origin. Available at: www.census.gov/population/www/projections/natsum-T3.html. Accessed May 8, 2007.

[2] Nelson EA, Dannefer D. Aged heterogeneity: fact or fiction? The fate of diversity in gerontological research. Gerontologist 1992;32(1):17–23.

[3] Evans CA, Kleinman DV. The Surgeon General's report on America's oral health: opportunities for the dental profession. J Am Dent Assoc 2000;13(12):1721–8.

[4] Ettinger RL. Restoring the aging dentition: repair of replacement. Int Dent J 1990;40(5):275–82.

[5] Ettinger RL, Mulligan R. The future of dental care for the elderly population. Calif Dent Assoc J 1999;27(9):687–92.

[6] Ettinger RL. Cohort differences among aging populations: a challenge for the dental profession. Spec Care Dentist 1993;13(1):19–26.

[7] Eklund SA. Changing treatment patterns. J Am Dent Assoc 1999;130(12):1707–12.

[8] Petersen PE, Yamamoto T. Improving the oral health of older people: the approach of the WHO Global Oral Health Programme. Community Dent Oral Epidemiol 2005;33:81–92.

[9] Cunha-Cruz J, Hujoel PP, Nadanovsky P. Secular trends in socio-economic disparities in edentulism: USA 1972–2001. J Dent Res 2007;86(2):131–6.

[10] CDC. Trends in oral health status: United States, 1988–1994 and 1999–2004. Vital Health Stat 11 2007;(248).

[11] Centers for Disease Control and Prevention. Total tooth loss among persons aged > 65 years—selected states, 1995–1997. MMWR Morb Mortal Wkly Rep 1999;48:206–10.

[12] MMWR Morb Mortal Wkly Rep 2003;52(50):1226–9.

[13] Jones DB, Niendorff WJ, Broderick EB. A review of the oral health of American Indian and Alaska Native elders. J Public Health Dent 2000;60(Suppl 1):256–60.

[14] Dolan TA, Atchison K, Huynh TN. Access to dental care among older adults in the United States. J Dent Educ 2005;69(9):961–74.

[15] Ettinger RL, Beck JD. Geriatric dental curriculum and the needs of the elderly. Spec Care Dent 1984;4(5):207–13.

[16] Jablonski RA, Munro CL, Grap MJ, et al. The role of biobehavioral, environmental, and social forces on oral health disparities in frail and functionally dependent nursing home elders. Biol Res Nurs 2005;7(1):75–82.

[17] Oral health in America: a report of the surgeon general. Rockville (MD): National Institute of Dental and Craniofacial Research; 2000.

[18] Ship J. Oral health in the elderly—what's missing? Oral Surg Oral Med Oral Pathol Oral Radiol Endod 2004;98(6):625–6.

[19] Dolan TA, Atchison KA. Implications of access, utilization and need for oral health care by the non-institutionalized and institutionalized elderly on the dental delivery system. J Dent Educ 1993;57(12):876–87.

[20] Berkey D, Berg R. Geriatric oral health issues in the United States. Int Dent J 2001; 51(Suppl 3):254–64.

[21] Evans C. Eliminating oral health disparities: ethics workshop reactor comments. J Dent Educ 2006;70(11):1180–3.

[22] Locker D. Does dental care improve the oral health of older adults? Comm Dent Health 2001;18(1):7–15.

[23] Barmes DE. Public policy on oral health and old age: a global view. J Public Health Dent 2000;60(4):335–7.

[24] National Health Interview Survey—Health United States 2006, Series 10, No.232, p. 96, 328–329.

[25] Kiyak HA. Measuring psychosocial variables that predict older persons' oral health behavior. Gerodontology 1996;13(2):69–75.

[26] Manski RJ, Moeller JF. Use of dental services. An analysis of visits, procedures and providers 1996. J Am Dent Assoc 2002;133(2):167–75.

[27] Gambucci JR, Martens LV, Meskin LH, et al. Dental care utilization patterns of older adults. Gerodontics 1986;2(1):11–5.

[28] Meskin LH, Dillenberg J, Heft MW, et al. Economic impact of dental service utilization by older adults. J Am Dent Assoc 1990;120(6):665–8.

[29] Kiyak HA, Reichmuth M. Barriers to and enablers of older adults' use of dental services. J Dent Educ 2005;69(9):975–86.

[30] Rudd R, Horowitz AM. The role of health literacy in achieving oral health for elders. J Dent Educ 2005;69(9):1018–21.

[31] Braun RJ, Marcus M. Comparing treatment decisions for elderly and young dental patients. Gerodontics 1985;1(3):138–42.

[32] Brown E, Manski R. Research findings #20: dental services: use, expenses, and sources of payment, 1996–2000. Rockville (MD): Agency for Healthcare Research and Quality; 2004.

[33] Robbertz AA, Lauf RC, Rupp RL, et al. A qualitative assessment of dental care access and utilization among the older adult population in the United States. Gen Dent 2006;54(5): 361–5.

[34] Rubinstein HG. Access to oral health care for elders: mere words or action? J Dent Educ 2005;69(9):1051–7.

[35] Dunlop DD, Manheim LM, Song J, et al. Gender and ethnic/racial disparities in health care utilization among older adults. J Gerontol B Psychol Sci Soc Sci 2002;57(4):S221–33.

[36] Pyle MA, Stoller EP. Oral health disparities among the elderly: interdisciplinary challenges for the future. J Dent Educ 2003;67(12):1327–36.

[37] Nunez B, Chalmers JM, Warren JJ. Provision of dental care for Iowa nursing homes. Spec Care Dent 2007, submitted.

[38] Altieri JP, Bruce SM, Crall JJ, et al. Future of dentistry. Today's vision: tomorrow's reality. J Am Dent Assoc 2002;133:1408–24.

[39] Anderson M. Prepaid dental annuity for retirement. J Dent Educ 2005;69(9):1032–3.

[40] Ettinger RL. Management of elderly patients in the private practice system. Int Dent J 1993; 43(1):29–40.

[41] Lee EE, Thomas CA, Vu T. Mobile and portable dentistry: alternative treatment services for the elderly. Spec Care Dentist 2001;21(4):153–5.

[42] Charlton DG, Ehrlich AD, Miniotis NJ. Current update on portable dental equipment. Compend Contin Educ Dent 2007;28(2):104–8.

[43] Association of State and Territorial Dental Directors. Mobile-portable dental manual. Available at: http://www.mobile-portabledentalmanual.com/. Accessed August 14, 2007.

[44] Chalmers JM. Oral health promotion for our ageing population. Aust Dent J 2003;48(1):2–9.

[45] Watt RG, Fuller S, Harnett R, et al. Oral health promotion evaluation—time for development. Comm Dent Oral Epidemiol 2001;29:161–6.

[46] Chalmers JM, Gryst M, Jolly M. Dental resource handbook. Adelaide, South Australia: The Alzheimer's Association of South Australia; 1997 [updated 2001].

[47] Ettinger RL. Rational dental care: part 1. Has the concept changed in 20 years? J Can Dent Assoc 2006;72(5):441–5.

[48] Chalmers JM. Minimal intervention dentistry: strategies for the new caries challenge in our older patients. J Can Dent Assoc 2006;72(5):325–31.

[49] Mohammad AR, Preshaw PM, Ettinger RL. Current status of predoctoral geriatric education in US dental schools. J Dent Educ 2003;67(5):509–14.

[50] Ettinger RL, McLeran H, Jakobsen J. Effect of a geriatric educational experience on graduates activities and attitudes. J Dent Educ 1990;54(5):273–8.

[51] Fabiano JA, Waldrop DP, Nochasjski TH, et al. Understanding dental students' knowledge and perceptions of older people: toward a new model of geriatric dental education. J Dent Educ 2005;69(4):419–33.

[52] Vargas C, Kramarow EA, Yellowitz JA. The oral health of older Americans. Centers for disease control and prevention. Aging Trends 2001;(3):1–8.

[53] Anusavice KJ. Dental caries: risk assessment and treatment solutions for an elderly population. Compend Contin Educ Dent 2002;23(Suppl 10):12–20.

[54] Chan DC, Wefel JS, Caughman WF. Practical fluoride and remineralization protocols for adult patients. Singapore Dent J 2004;26(1):1–6.

[55] Gooch BF, Malvitz DM, Griffin SO, et al. Promoting the oral health of older adults through the chronic disease model: CDC's perspective on what we still need to know. J Dent Educ 2005;69(9):1058–63.

[56] Pearson A, Chalmers JM. Oral hygiene care for adults with dementia in residential aged care facilities. a systematic review. JBI Reports 2004;2(3):65–113.

[57] Lynch E, Baysan A. Reversal of primary root caries using a dentifrice with a high fluoride content. Caries Res 2001;35(Suppl 1):60–4.

[58] Weintraub JA. Fluoride varnish for caries prevention: comparisons with other preventive agents and recommendations for a community-based protocol. Spec Care Dentist 2003; 23(5):180–6.

[59] American Dental Association Council on Scientific Affairs. Professionally applied topical fluoride: evidence-based clinical recommendations. J Dent Educ 2007;71(3):393–402.

[60] Brailsford SR, Fiske J, Gilbert S, et al. The effects of the combination of chlorhexidine/thymol- and fluoride-containing varnishes on the severity of root caries lesions in frail institutionalised elderly people. J Dent 2002;30(7–8):319–24.

[61] Banting DW, Papas A, Clark DC, et al. The effectiveness of 10% chlorhexidine varnish treatment on dental caries incidence in adults with dry mouth. Gerodontology 2000;17(2): 67–76.

[62] Wyatt CC, MacEntee MI. Caries management for institutionalized elders using fluoride and chlorhexidine mouthrinses. Comm Dent Oral Epid 2004;32(5):322–8.

[63] Clavero J, Baca P, Junco P, et al. Effects of a 0.2% chlorhexidine spray applied once or twice daily on plaque accumulation and gingival inflammation in a geriatric population. J Clin Periodontal 2003;30(9):773–7.

[64] Hay KD, Thomson WM. A clinical trial of the anticaries efficacy of casein derivatives complexed with calcium phosphate. Oral Surg Oral Med Oral Pathol Oral Radiol Endod 2002; 93:271–5.

[65] Cross KJ, Huq NL, Reynolds EC. Casein phosphopeptides in oral health—chemistry and clinical applications. Curr Pharm Des 2007;13(8):793–800.

[66] Walsh LJ. Chapter 7: Lifestyle impacts on oral health. In: Mount GJ, Hume WR, editors. Preservation and restoration of tooth structure. Sandgate (Qld): Knowledge Books and Software; 2005.

[67] Epstein JB, Emerton S, Le ND, et al. A double-blind crossover trial of Oral Balance gel and Biotene toothpaste versus placebo in patents with xerostomia following radiation therapy. Oral Oncol 1999;35:132–7.

[68] Hay KD, Morton RP. The efficacy of casein phosphoprotein-calcium phosphate complex (DC-CP) [Dentacal^{RTM}] as a mouth moistener in patients with severe xerostomia. N Z Dent J 2003;99:46–8.

[69] MacEntee MI, Thorne S, Kazanjian A. Conflicting priorities: oral health in long-term care. Spec Care Dentist 1999;19:164–72.

[70] MacEntee MI. Oral care for successful aging in long term care. J Public Health Dent 2000;60: 326–9.

[71] Ettinger RL, Watkins C, Cowen H. Reflections on changes in geriatric dentistry. J Dent Educ 2000;64:715–22.

[72] Chalmers JM, Levy SM, Buckwalter KC, et al. Factors influencing nurses aides' provision of oral care for nursing facility residents. Spec Care Dent 1996;16(2):71–9.

[73] Pyfferoen M, Cody K, Chalmers J, et al. Observation of mealtime and oral hygiene cares for dementia residents [abstract 0955]. New Orleans (LA): IADR; 2007.

[74] Bowers BJ, Esmond S, Jacobson N. The relationship between staffing and quality in long-term care facilities: exploring views of nurses aides. J Nurs Care Qual 2000;14:55–64.

[75] Coleman P, Watson NM. Oral care provided by certified nursing assistants in nursing homes. J Am Ger Soc 2006;54(1):138–43.

[76] Pennington K, Scott J, Magilvy K. The role of certified nursing assistants in nursing homes. J Nurs Adm 2003;33(11):578–84.

[77] Simons D, Baker P, Jones B, et al. An evaluation of an oral health training programme for carers of the elderly in residential homes. Br Dent J 2000;188(4):206–10.

[78] Nicol R, Petrina Sweeney M, McHugh S, et al. Effectiveness of health care worker training on the oral health of elderly residents of nursing homes. Comm Dent Oral Epid 2005;33(2): 115–24.

[79] Frenkel HF. Behind the screens: care staff observations on delivery of oral health care in nursing homes. Gerodontology 1999;16:75–80.

[80] Frenkel H, Harvey I, Newcombe RG. Improving oral health institutionalized elderly people by educating caregivers: a randomized controlled trial. Community Dent Oral Epidemiol 2001;29:289–97.

[81] Frenkel H, Harvey I, Needs K. Oral health care education and its effect on caregivers' knowledge and attitudes: a randomized controlled trial. Community Dent Oral Epidemiol 2002;30: 91–100.

[82] Wyatt CL, So FHC, Williams PM, et al. The development, implementation, utilization and outcomes of a comprehensive dental program for older adults residing in long-term care facilities. J Can Dent Assoc 2006;72(5):419–27.

[83] Chalmers JM. 2007 IGEC-CNA training module. Available at: http://www.healthcare. uiowa.edu/igec/e-learn_cert/modules_intro/default.asp. Accessed June 6, 2007.

[84] Kayser-Jones J, Bird WF, Paul SM, et al. An instrument to assess the oral health status of nursing home residents. Gerontologist 1995;35:814–24.

[85] Chalmers JM, King PL, Spencer AJ, et al. The oral health assessment tool—validity and reliability. Aust Dent J 2005;50(3):191–9.

[86] Chalmers JM. 2007 IGEC-OHAT training module. Available at: http://www.healthcare. uiowa.edu/igec/e-learn_lic/dentistry/default.asp. Accessed June 6, 2007.

ELSEVIER
SAUNDERS

THE DENTAL
CLINICS
OF NORTH AMERICA

Dent Clin N Am 52 (2008) 447–461

Improving and Maintaining Oral Health for People with Special Needs

Paul Glassman, DDS, MA, MBA*, Paul Subar, DDS

University of the Pacific, Arthur A. Dugoni School of Dentistry, 2155 Webster Street, San Francisco, CA 94115, USA

Who are people with special needs?

There are many terms that have been used to describe people who have trouble receiving dental treatment in a routine manner. These include "people with special needs," "children with special health care needs," "people with disabilities," and "people with complex needs," among other terms [1–3]. Some of these terms, such as "children with special health care needs" or people with "developmental disabilities" have definitions that are found in federal regulations and used for collection of data and funding purposes [4,5]. Other terms, such as "people with special needs" or "people with disabilities" do not have generally agreed upon definitions, although they are widely used and useful in describing populations who afford challenges in providing oral health services. For the purpose of this clinically focused article, the terms "people with special needs" and "people with disabilities" will be used interchangeably, and a broad definition of these terms will be used: people who have difficulty accessing dental treatment services because of complicated medical, physical, social, or psychologic conditions [6]. This article discusses the implications for the oral health profession, given an expanding population of people with special needs, describes the challenges of providing oral health services for this population, and discusses the implications of these challenges for the organization of the oral health delivery system.

The population of people with special needs is increasing dramatically

The number of people with special needs who need oral health services is rising dramatically. The United States Census reported in 2000 that 49.7

---

* Corresponding author.
E-mail address: pglassman@pacific.edu (P. Glassman).

million people in the United States population had a long-standing condition or disability [7]. They represented 19.3% of 257.2 million people who were aged 5 and older in the civilian noninstitutionalized population, or nearly one person in five. Fig. 1 illustrates that the major areas of disability are physical, sensory, and mental disabilities, as well as difficulty going outside. A significant portion of the population, 9.5% of those over age 65, also have problems with basic self care. Also of interest in the 2000 census data was the finding that 46.3% of people with at least one disability reported having more than one diability.

There is an extensive body of literature that demonstrates that people with disabilities have more dental disease, more missing teeth, and more difficulty obtaining dental care than other members of the general population [8–12]. People with developmental disabilities who reside in community settings have significant unmet medical and dental needs [13–20]. The situation is worse for individuals with disabilities who live in rural areas [21].

Percentage of the Civilian Noninstitutionalized Population With a Disability by Age and Type of Disability: 2000

(For more information on confidentiality protection, sampling error, nonsampling error, and definitions, see *www.census.gov/prod/cen2000/doc/sf3.pdf*)

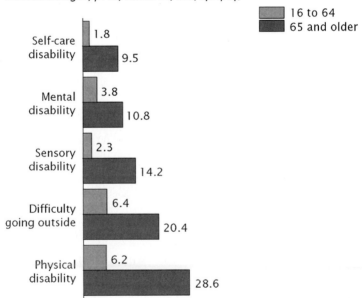

Source: U.S. Census Bureau, Census 2000 Summary File 3.

Fig. 1. Population with disabilities by age and type of disability. (*Data from* US Census Bureau, Census 2000 Summary File 3.)

The Surgeon General's Report on Oral Health points out that people with mental retardation (MR) or other developmental disabilities have significantly higher rates of poor oral hygiene and an increased need for periodontal treatment than the general population [2]. People with disabilities also have a higher rate of dental caries than the general population, and almost two thirds of community-based residential facilities report having inadequate access to dental care [22–24] [Dwyer, Northern Wisconsin Center for the Developmentally Disabled, unpublished data, 1996]. Untreated dental disease has been found in at least 25% of people with cerebral palsy, 30% of those with head injuries, and 17% of those with hearing impairment [8]. A study commissioned by the Special Olympics concluded that individuals with MR have poorer oral health, more untreated caries, and a higher prevalence of gingivitis and other periodontal diseases than the general population [25].

In 1999 the United States Special Olympics Special Smiles Program performed extremely conservative oral assessments (no x-rays, mirrors, or explorers) of athletes of all ages, and found that 13% of the athletes reported some form of oral pain, 39% demonstrated signs of gingival infection, and nearly 25% had untreated decay [Oral health status and needs of Special Olympics athletes—world summer games, Raleigh, North Carolina: June 26 – July 4, 1999. Special Olympics International, unpublished report, 1999]. These findings are in a population that tends to be from higher-income families. However, people from lower socio-economic groups and those covered by Medicaid also have more dental disease and receive fewer dental services than the general population, and many individuals with disabilities are in these lower socio-economic groups [2,26,27].

The number of people with disabilities living in communities and seeking oral health care is also impacted by the movement toward deinstitutionalization. In the mid-20th century, many people with physical and mental disabilities were institutionalized and institution-based preventive dentistry programs were developed [28–30]. However, since the 1970s, almost two-thirds of those residing in institutional settings have been moved into community-based settings, and dental care services, which had been available in the institution, are in many cases no longer unavailable for them [31]. The idea that these individuals would be able to access generic oral health services available in the community has turned out to be wishful thinking not matched by reality. Annually, 36.5% of people 15 years and older and classified as severely disabled, reported a dental visit, compared with 53.4% of those with no disability [27]. Few states cover dental services for adults under Medicaid. Even in those states with Medicaid coverage, low reimbursement rates and the reluctance of practitioners to accept those rates, reduces the availability care—including hospitalization and anesthesia—required for treating patients with disabilities [8].

The limited availability of dental providers trained and willing to serve people with special needs, and limited third-party support for the delivery of complex services, further complicates the problem of limited access to oral health services [2]. Some believe that the United States health care system discriminates against people with disabilities because health care professionals are uncomfortable working with people with disabilities and find ways not to treat them [32].

The nation's aging adult population is especially at high risk for dental problems, particularly those elderly with health problems or other disabilities. An estimated 70% of the nation's 2-million-plus nursing home population has dental problems, including dentures that do not fit, loss of some or all of their teeth, and most significantly, poor oral hygiene [8]. Most people are aware of the "graying of America," the phrase used to describe the fact that the number of people in the United States population over 65 has increased more than tenfold from 1900 to 2000, and represents almost 13% of the total population [33]. These older adults are expected to grow to 70 million by 2030, when they will represent 20% of the population. Even more dramatic growth is expected in the number of people over the age of 85, which will reach 19 million by 2050, representing 5% of the total population. Fig. 2 illustrates the increase in the population over 65 and 85 in the coming decades. This oldest old-age group is especially important for the future of our health care system, because these individuals tend to be in poorer health and require more services than the younger old-age group.

While most people are aware of the aging of the population, it is not widely understood that at the same time that the elderly population is increasing, the rate of edentulism is decreasing dramatically [2]. In California, only 13% of people over 65 are edentulous now, compared with close to 50% only a few decades ago. Fig. 3 illustrates the dramatic drop in the

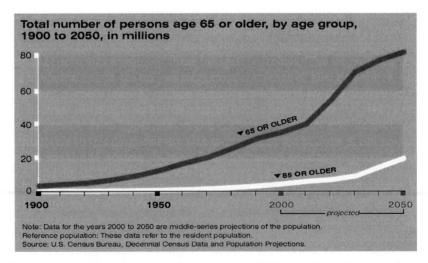

Fig. 2. Growth in the elderly population. (*Data from* US Census Bureau, Decennial Census Data and Population Projections.)

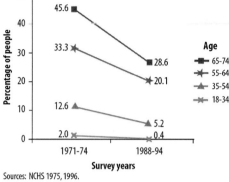

Fig. 3. Rate of edentulism in United States population. (*Data from* National Center for Health Statistics, 1975, 1996.)

edentulism rate from the early 1970s to the 1990s. This new population of "baby boomers with teeth" has invested heavily in maintaining oral health, has complex restorations that require maintenance, and will present significant challenges to the dental profession, as they become less able to maintain good oral health.

The economic burden of oral disease in people with disabilities

Oral health professionals who work with populations of individuals are aware of many instances where untreated oral disease in people with disabilities resulted in pain, suffering, high medical costs, and even death [34]. For example, in Louisiana in 2003, a $70 extraction would have saved an elderly patient 15 days in the hospital, including 2 days in an intensive care unit, and a $35,000 medical bill [35]. In California, a young autistic lady who was nonverbal began to act out and hit other residents of her community residential care facility. She was admitted to a locked psychiatric facility at a cost of $150,000 per year to the State of California. Fortunately, it was eventually discovered that she had dental problems. Once her dental problems were treated, her aggressive behaviors ceased and she was able to return to her community. The Pacific Center for Special Care at the University of the Pacific, Arthur A. Dugoni School of Dentistry produced a moving video of these events [36].

The vast majority of adults with disabilities are low income and very few states provide Medicaid dental benefits [34]. There is evidence that people without sources of dental care turn to costly emergency room services and subsequent hospitalizations [37,38]. There is also a growing body of literature on the association between oral disease and systemic health conditions.

These conditions include heart disease, premature birth and low birth weight infants, nursing home acquired pneumonia, diabetes, and stroke [39–51].

People with disabilities have the highest incidence of general health problems in our society. In fact, it has been calculated that providing oral health benefits for the population of people defined under Medicaid as being "aged, blind, or disabled" would save enough money in Medicare and Medicaid general health costs to entirely pay for a national system of Medicaid oral health benefits [34].

Challenges in providing oral health care for people with disabilities

There are numerous challenges in providing oral health services for people with special needs that go beyond the normal considerations for other populations. These challenges require oral health professionals to have extraordinary training, empathy, patience, and desire to be successful. There are a number of areas where providing oral health services for these populations presents unique challenges.

First, there is a need to understand and to be prepared to work with people with a wide variety of general health conditions. While oral health professionals do not need to have complete knowledge of every general health condition that their patients present with, it is essential that they have the knowledge and experience to gather and apply the information they need. This implies the training and ability to function in health care teams and get consultations from physicians, social workers, and other general and social service professionals.

There is also a need for oral health professionals to understand the social service systems that operate in their community and the social context in which oral health services take place. They need to understand community living arrangements, social service agencies, and advocacy organizations operating in their community. They also need to understand the appropriate use of language when interacting with individuals with special needs and their caregivers. There is a growing movement advocating the use of "People First" language [52–54]. This language emphasizes the fact that disability is a part of the human condition and all people want to be described by their abilities rather than labeled by their disabilities. An oral health professional who does not understand this language, and refers to people he or she treats as "the handicapped patients I see," risks alienating the individual, their caregiver, and those advocating for full inclusion in our society.

Oral health professionals also need to understand the extraordinary vulnerability of people with special needs to abuse and neglect in our society [55,56]. They need to understand how to recognize abuse and neglect and their role as mandated reporters. Oral health providers are health professionals, and as a part of the health care team they may find that their patients are depressed, suicidal, or unable to cope with various living challenges. They have an obligation to intervene, provide basic diagnosis and counseling, and make appropriate referrals for follow-up of these situations.

Oral health professionals need to understand how to prevent oral diseases in people with various disabilities. There are special challenges presented by working with someone where communication and even procedures need to be performed by a third person, the caregiver. Some people have limited physical ability to perform oral hygiene procedures, and "partial participation" programs need to be designed and performed. This term refers to having the individual do as much as they are able to, but having a caregiver ensure that needed prevention procedures are completed. There are numerous informational, physical, and behavioral obstacles to be addressed. These are described in detail in a caregiver training package titled "Overcoming Obstacles to Dental Health," a training package for caregivers of people with disabilities [57]. In addition to this package, there is a large amount of literature that describes the challenges and techniques for helping people with special needs prevent oral diseases [6,58–60].

Oral health professionals need to be familiar with a variety of treatment options for providing oral health services for people with special needs. Fig. 4 describes some of the modalities that are available to help people have dental services performed. The modalities on the left side of the continuum are those with the least expense and side effects. Oral health professionals who are in the best position to provide treatment using the optimal modality for the individual they are seeing are the professionals who have all these options available personally or by referral. For example, if there are no dental offices where behavioral or physical supports are provided in a given community, then more people may end up having dental treatment via sedation or general anesthesia than is necessary.

In addition to understanding and having various treatment options available, oral health professionals also need to consider a wide variety of factors

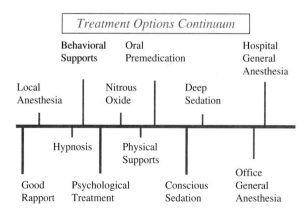

Fig. 4. Treatment options continuum. (*Courtesy of* P. Glassman, DDS, MA, MBA, San Francisco, CA.)

when developing a treatment plan for an individual with special needs. In addition to those factors already mentioned, there can also be limitations in an individual's understanding and physical ability to obtain needed services. Some oral problems are exacerbated by medical problems, side effects of medication, or by the disability itself [2].

Fig. 5 illustrates a schema for gathering data that starts with information about the individual's medical, physical, and psychologic condition, and includes social and personal information as well as dental information. Although every dental professional student has learned the components of a complete health history, the nondental aspects of this data gathering process can be neglected for some patients. These components of the history are essential for a person with a complex condition.

Also note that in Fig. 5 the data gathering process leads to a diagnosis, and ultimately a treatment plan with four components or four treatment plans. These essential aspects of treatment planning for people with special needs are illustrated in Fig. 6. Often, oral health professionals condense these components into a single plan. However, when planning dental treatment for an individual with a complex situation, it is critical that each of these elements be considered and planned separately. Special consideration should be given to the prevention plan. This part of the plan is actually a diagnostic step, as it is critical to understand the degree that prevention practices can be put into place for this individual before a decision is made about other treatment.

It is also critical to consider a long-term plan for this individual before deciding on a course of initial treatment. This involves a careful analysis of the person's medical, physical, social, and psychologic conditions, and an analysis of the prognosis of these factors in combination with their oral conditions. For example, it would be inadvisable to construct a complex dental prosthesis that requires meticulous care for an individual who has a neurodegenerative disorder that will predictably result in a significant

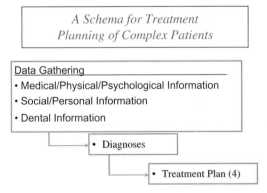

Fig. 5. Treatment planning schema. (*Courtesy of* P. Glassman, DDS, MA, MBA, San Francisco, CA.)

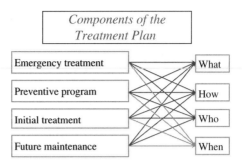

Fig. 6. Components of the treatment plan. (*Courtesy of* P. Glassman, DDS, MA, MBA, San Francisco, CA.)

physical decline and death over the next 3 or 4 years. Finally, for each of the four treatment plans it is critical to consider what will be done, how it will be accomplished, who will be responsible for doing it, and when it will be undertaken.

Training of oral health professionals

Surveys of dentists, that contain questions about the perceived preparation of dentists to treat people with special needs, have indicated that most general dentists do not feel adequately prepared to treat people with moderate or severe medical, behavioral, or physical problems (Glassman, unpublished data, 2001, 2006). This factor is a part of the rationale for the repeated call for a required year of postdoctoral education following graduation from dental school, and study of the feasibility of such a requirement [61–69]. In spite of this recommendation by numerous national commissions, a postdoctoral year of training is required in only two states: Delaware and New York.

A recent revision of the Accreditation Standards for Dental Education Programs by the Commission on Dental Accreditation (CODA) added a new standard, 2-26, which states that "Graduates must be competent in assessing the treatment needs of patients with special needs" [70]. There is no requirement that graduates have any experience treating people with special needs during their education program. Furthermore, there are only enough postdoctoral general dentistry training programs to enroll about 25% of dental graduates, so the majority of general dentists enter practice with little or no experience in treating this population.

In 2005, the American Dental Education House of Delegates adopted a resolution calling on CODA to "adopt accreditation standards that ensure that education programs include both didactic instruction and clinical experiences involving treatment of people with special needs as defined by the Commission, and appropriate for the type of educational program in which the student is enrolled" [71]. There is still no requirement in the accreditation standards for dental education programs that graduates have any experience treating people with special needs, in spite of this resolution.

Implications for the oral health system

The dramatic population shifts and the increased level of expertise described above are presenting increasing challenges for the oral health care system. This article has presented some of the many reasons why the oral health of people with special needs is poorer than the general population and access to dental services is more restricted. The current oral health care system is not working well for those populations. Increasing oral health workforce shortages, inadequate training of oral health professionals, and a reimbursement system which does not reward the kinds of services needed by these populations all contribute to the failure of the current system for these groups. This is compounded by the fact that the current system of care relies predominantly on dental offices and clinics to provide all levels of oral health services, including screening, oral health education, minor procedures, and complex procedures. A dental office or clinic may not be the only place where some of these services can be provided, and for some services it may not be the best place. In particular, preventive services may be more effectively delivered in settings closer to where people live and spend the majority of their time. In addition, there is little integration in the United States between the oral health system and general health and social service systems, which are in regular contact with people with disabilities. As described above, the result is significant oral health disparities with more dental disease, few preventive services, and significant access problems for people with special needs.

In 2004 a conference sponsored by the Pacific Center for Special Care at the University of the Pacific School of Dentistry and the Special Care Dentistry Association concluded that this situation is likely to get worse over time rather than better [3]. The purpose of this conference was to explore the changing population of people with special needs, analyze the implications for the dental profession and society, and describe systems and strategies that might lead to improved oral health for these populations. The consensus statement from that conference recommends a number of steps that need to be taken to reform the oral health delivery system so it can be responsive to the needs of people with disabilities. The statement describes characteristics of a new system that might better address the oral health of people with disabilities. These include:

A focus on prevention
An incentive system that addresses services likely to improve oral health for these populations
A system integrated with other community health and social service systems

A case management approach, where oral diseases can be identified and people referred to care settings that best match their situation and needs

A tiered delivery system, with oral health professionals serving as coaches, mentors, and supporters of other health and social service professionals

A system that engages caregivers closest to the individual in playing a major role in maintaining oral health

A tiered delivery system, where increasingly complex care is performed by those with the most extensive training to deliver such care, and less complex care is delivered by those with less extensive training

There are a number of trends and proposals that have been developed to address some of the issues listed above. One of these is the expansion of the scope of duties of dental hygienists. A 2004 study released by the Health Resources and Services Administration stated that in 2001 there were 22 states where current or pending regulations allowed dental hygienists to practice in expanded settings or with reduced supervision [72]. In addition, these are new workforce models being proposed by the American Dental Association (ADA) and the American Dental Hygienists Association (ADHA). Both of these major oral health organizations cite the problems with access by people with special needs as central to the reason they have developed these proposals. The ADA has proposed a Community Dental Health Coordinator (CDHC), while the ADHA has proposed an Advanced Dental Hygiene Practitioner (ADHP) [73,74]. Both of these models are along the continuum of a community health worker. Many types of community health workers are employed in the United States health care system and there is evidence that they can increase access to care for underserved populations [75]. There is a continuum of background for community health workers with the "promotora" (health promoter from the community) being at the lay person, community member, and end of the continuum [76]. The ADHA's ADHP proposal is at the opposite end, with the position described as requiring masters level training beyond the dental hygiene degree and involving the performance of technical dental procedures. The ADA's CDHC proposal is closer to the lay person end of the scale, with the proposal that this position could be filled by someone with a high school education and a year or less of additional community health and oral health training.

While it is not clear how these specific proposals will evolve, it is clear that there is widespread support for new kinds of oral health providers that can extend the reach of the current oral health workforce beyond the walls of traditional dental offices and clinics. It is likely that there will be a number of experiments in the coming decade, with various workforce models and alternate delivery systems to better serve currently underserved populations, including people with disabilities and other special needs.

There are also proposals about increased financing for oral health services for low-income persons with disabilities. The Special Care Dentistry

Act, introduced in 2005, would provide for adult Medicaid benefits in every state for low-income individuals who are "aged, blind, or disabled." An analysis of the rationale and cost of this measure indicated that it would cost less that 0.5% of the national expenditures under Medicare and Medicaid, and would be likely to reduce expenditures for those programs in excess of the cost [34].

Summary

The number of people in the United States population with disabilities and other special needs is growing dramatically. These individuals present unique challenges for oral health professionals in planning and carrying out dental treatment, and for the oral health delivery system. It has been recognized that the current delivery system is not working well for these populations. New workforce, financing, and delivery models are beginning to emerge that may hold promise for creating and maintaining oral health for currently underserved populations, including people with disabilities and other special needs.

References

[1] Waldman HB, Perlman SP, Waldman HB, et al. Children with special health care needs: results of a national survey. J Dent Child 2006;73(1):57–62.

[2] U.S. Department of Health and Human Services. Oral Health in America: a Report of the Surgeon General. Rockville (MD): U.S. Department of Health and Human Services, National Institute of Dental and Craniofacial Research, National Institutes of Health; 2000.

[3] Glassman P, Henderson T, Helgeson M, et al. Consensus statement: oral health for people with special needs: consensus statement on implications and recommendations for the dental profession. J Calif Dent Assoc 2005;33(8):619–23.

[4] Newacheck PW, Rising JP, Kim SE. Children at risk for special health care needs. Pediatrics 2007;118(1):334–42.

[5] Definition of Developmental Disability. 42 US Code, Section 15002(8). 1978.

[6] Glassman P, Anderson M, Jacobsen P, et al. Practical protocols for the prevention of dental disease in community settings for people with special needs: the protocols. Spec Care Dentist 2003;23(5):160–4.

[7] U.S. Department of Commerce, Economics and Statistics Administration, U.S. Census Bureau. Census 2000 Brief. Disability Status 2000. March 2003.

[8] The Disparity Cavity: filling America's oral health gap. Oral Health America, May 2000.

[9] Haavio ML. Oral health care of the mentally retarded and other persons with disabilities in the Nordic countries: present situation and plans for the future. Spec Care Dentist 1995;15: 65–9.

[10] Feldman CA, Giniger M, Sanders M, et al. Special Olympics, special smiles: assessing the feasibility of epidemiologic data collection. J Am Dent Assoc 1997;128:1687–96.

[11] Waldman HB, Perlman SP, Swerdloff M. Use of pediatric dental services in the 1990s: some continuing difficulties. J Dent Child 2000;67:59–63.

[12] Oral Health: Factors Contributing to Low Use of Dental Services by Low-Income Populations. United States General Accounting Office. Report to Congressional Requesters. September 2000.

[13] Minihan PM, Dean DH. Meeting the needs for health services of persons with mental retardation living in the community. Aust J Polit Hist 1990;80:1043–8.

[14] Schor EL, Smalky KA, Neff JM. Primary care of previously institutionalized retarded children. Pediatrics 1981;67:536–40.

[15] McDonald EP. Medical needs of severely developmentally disabled persons residing in the community. Am J Ment Defic 1985;90:171–6.

[16] Ziring PR, Kastner T, Friedman DL, et al. Provision of health care for persons with developmental disabilities living in the community. JAMA 1988;260:1439–44.

[17] Dane JN. The Missouri Elks Mobile Dental Program—dental care for developmentally disabled persons. J Public Health Dent 1990;50:42–7.

[18] Preest M, Gelber S. Dental health and treatment of a group of physically handicapped adults. Community Health 1977;9:29–34.

[19] Ferguson FS, Kamen P, Ratner S, et al. Dental fellowships in developmental disabilities help broaden care of the disabled. NY State Dent J 1992;58(9):55–8.

[20] Wilson KI. Treatment accessibility for physically and mentally handicapped people—a review of the literature. Community Dent Health 1992;9:187–92.

[21] Hill EG. Health Care in Rural California: the 1990–91 budget from Perspectives and Issues, Reports of the Legislative Analyst. Legislative Analyst's Office, Sacramento California, 1990.

[22] Beck JD, Hunter RJ. Oral health status in the United States: problems of special patients. J Dent Educ 1985;149:407–25.

[23] White BA, Caplan DJ, Weintraub JA. A quarter century of changes in oral health in the United States. J Dent Educ 1995;59(1):19–60.

[24] Waldman HB, Perlman SP, Swerdloff M. What if dentists did not treat people with disabilities? J Dent Child 1998;65:96–101.

[25] Horwitz S, Kerker B, Owens P, et al. The health status and needs of individuals with mental retardation. Special Olympics 2000. Available at: http://www.specialolympics. org/Special+Olympics+Public+Website/English/Initiatives/Research/Health_Research/ Health+Status+and+Needs.htm. Accessed December 2, 2007.

[26] U.S. Bureau of the Census: Americans with disabilities: 1994–95. Current Population reports. P70–61. Census Brief, CENBR/97–5 Washington DC: U.S. Department of Commerce, Economics and Statistics Administration; 1997b Dec.

[27] Stiefel DJ. Adults with Disabilities. Dental Care Considerations of Disadvantages and Special Care Populations: proceedings of the Conference Held April 18–19, 2001, in Baltimore, Maryland. U.S. Department of Health and Human Services, Health Resources and Services Administration, Bureau of Health Professions, Division of Medicine and Dentistry, Division of Nursing. April 2001.

[28] Kass L. Dental care programs for the institutionally mentally retarded. Dent Hyg 1979;53: 76–8.

[29] Full CA, Kerber PE, Boender P, et al. Oral health maintenance of the institutionalized handicapped child. J Am Dent Assoc 1977;94(1):111–3.

[30] Udin R, Kuster C. The influence of motivation on a plaque control program for handicapped children. J Am Dent Assoc 1984;109:591–3.

[31] Thornton JB, al-Zahid S, Campbell V, et al. Oral hygiene levels and periodontal disease prevalence among residents with mental retardation at various residential settings. Spec Care Dentist 1989;9(6):186–90.

[32] Schriver T. Testimony before a Special Hearing of a Subcommittee of the Committee On Appropriations of the United States Senate One Hundred Seventh Congress, First Session. Anchorage, Alaska. March 5, 2001.

[33] Federal Interagency Forum on Aging Related Statistics. Older Americans 2000: Key Indicators of Well Being. 2000.

[34] Glassman P, Folse G. Financing oral health services for people with special needs: projecting national expenditures. J Calif Dent Assoc 2005;33(9):731–40.

[35] Folse G. Oral health shame: a call to action. Exceptional parent magazine 2005;35(7):63.

[36] Pacific Center for Special Care. Sarah's story. A four-minute video describing Sarah's admission to a locked facility, dental treatment, and return to her community. Available at: http://www.pacificspecialcare.org/sarah.htm. Accessed September 1, 2007.

[37] Cohen LA, Manski RJ, Magder LS, et al. Dental visits to hospital emergency departments by adults receiving Medicaid: assessing their use. J Am Dent Assoc 2002;133(6):715–24.

[38] Cohen LA, Magder LS, Manski RJ, et al. Hospital admissions associated with nontraumatic dental emergencies in a Medicaid population. Am J Emerg Med 2003;21(7):540–4.

[39] Association of State and Territorial Health Officials. Health Focus. Medicaid: covering dental care could lower heart disease costs. Available at: http://www.statepublichealth.org/index.php?template=view_story.php&fs_id=16&PHPSESSID=592a584e08d591ae3f3f9e199360f1c7. Accessed June 13, 2005.

[40] Desvarieux M, Demmer RT, Rundek T, et al. Periodontal microbiota and carotid intima-media thickness. Circulation 2005;111:576–82.

[41] Desvarieux M, Demmer RT, Rundek T, et al. Relationship between periodontal disease, tooth loss, carotid artery plaque. Stroke 2003;34(9):2120–5.

[42] Hoyert DL, Arias E, Smith BL, et al. (2001). Deaths: final Data for 1999. National Center for Health Statistics. Monthly Vital Statistics Report, 49(8).

[43] Krol D, Edelstein B, De Biasi A. Periodontal disease association with poor birth outcomes: state of the science and policy implications. Children's Dental Health Project. June 4, 2003. Available at: http://www.cdhp.org/downloads/Publications/Policy/PTLBW.pdf. Accessed June 15, 2005.

[44] Offenbacher S, Beck J. Potential Impact of Maternal Periodontitis on Reproductive Outcomes. CDC Conference on Public Health Implications of Chronic Periodontal Infections in Adults. April 2003. Available at: http://www.cdc.gov/OralHealth/conferences/periodontal_infections12.htm. Accessed June 20, 2005.

[45] El-Solh AA, Pietrantoni C, Bhat A, et al. Colonization of dental plaques: a reservoir of respiratory pathogens for hospital-acquired pneumonia in institutionalized elders. Chest 2004;126:1575–82.

[46] Mealey B. American Academy of Periodontology position paper on diabetes and periodontal diseases. J Periodontol 2000;71:664–78.

[47] Genco R. Diabetes and Periodontal Disease: current concepts. CDC Conference on Public Health Implications of Chronic Periodontal Infections in Adults. April 2003. Available at: http://www.cdc.gov/OralHealth/conferences/periodontal_infections09.htm. Accessed June 20, 2005.

[48] White JE. Loss of dental support increases risk for ischemic stroke. J Am Osteopath Assoc 1999;99(10):502 [Letter].

[49] Grau AJ, Becher H, Ziegler CM, et al. Periodontal disease as a risk factor for ischemic stroke. Stroke 2004;35(2):496–501.

[50] Joshipura K. The relationship between oral conditions and ischemic stroke and peripheral vascular disease. J Am Dent Assoc 2002;133(Suppl):23S–30S.

[51] Genco R, Offenbacher S, Beck J. Periodontal disease and cardiovascular disease: epidemiology and possible mechanisms. J Am Dent Assoc 2002;133(Suppl):14S–22S.

[52] Snow K. People First Language. Available at: http://www.disabilityisnatural.com/peoplefirstlanguage.htm. Accessed September 1, 2007.

[53] West Virginians with Developmental Disabilities. People First Language. Available at: http://www.wvddc.org/people_first.html. Accessed September 1, 2007.

[54] The Life Span Institute. Guidelines for Reporting and Writing about People with Disabilities. Available at: http://www.lsi.ku.edu/lsi/internal/guidelines.html. Accessed September 1, 2007.

[55] Glassman P, Chavez E, Hawks D. Abuse and neglect of elderly individuals: guidelines for oral health professionals. J Calif Dent Assoc 2004;32(4):323–5.

[56] Glassman P, Miller C, Ingraham R, et al. The extraordinary vulnerability of people with disabilities: guidelines for oral health professionals. J Calif Dent Assoc 2004;32(5):379–86.

[57] Miller C, Glassman P, Wozniak T, et al. Overcoming Obstacles To Dental Health—A Training Program For Caregivers Of People With Disabilities. 4th edition. 1998.

[58] Glassman P, Miller C. Dental disease prevention and people with special needs. J Calif Dent Assoc 2003;31(2):149–60.

[59] Glassman P, Miller C. Preventing dental disease for people with special needs: the need for practical preventive protocols for use in community settings. Spec Care Dentist 2003;23(5): 165–7.

[60] Glassman P, Miller C. Effect of preventive dentistry training program for caregivers in community facilities on caregiver and client behavior and client oral hygiene. NY State Dent J 2006;72(2):38–46.

[61] VanOstenberg PR. Advanced general dentistry education programs: issues and forces that will shape the future. J Dent Educ 1983;47:364–8.

[62] American Dental Association. Special Committee on the Future of Dentistry. Strategic Plan. Issue Papers on Dental Research, Manpower, Education, Practice and Public and Professional Concerns and Recommendations for Action. July, 1983.

[63] Advanced Dental Education. Recommendations for the 80's. Issues in dental health policy series. WK Kellog Foundation. Washington, DC: American Association of Dental Schools; 1980.

[64] Special Issue. Symposium on required postdoctoral education programs in general dentistry. J Dent Educ 1987;51:273–321.

[65] American Association of Dental Schools. Proceedings of the 1992 House of Delegates, Resolution 11S-92-11. A year of postdoctoral study. J Dent Educ 1992;56:454–5.

[66] Field M, editor. Institute of medicine. Dental education at the crossroads: challenges and change. Washington D.C.: National Academy Press; 1995. p. 14.

[67] Formicola AJ, Myers R. A postdoctoral year for the practice of dentistry: rationale and progress. J Dent Educ 1991;55:526–30.

[68] American Association of Dental Schools. Proceedings of the 1994 House of Delegates. Expansion of postdoctoral general dentistry training: meeting national need and demand. J Dent Educ 1994;58:505–16.

[69] Shugars DA, O'Neil EH, Bader JD, editors. Healthy America: practitioners for 2005, an agenda for action for U.S. health professional schools. Durham (NC): The Pew Health Commission; 1991.

[70] American Dental Association. Commission on Dental Accreditation. Accreditation Standards for Dental Education Programs. 2007.

[71] American Dental Education Association House of Delegates. Resolution 18H-2004. March, 2005.

[72] HRSA. The Professional Practice Environment of Dental Hygienists in the Fifty States and the District of Columbia, 2001. April 2004.

[73] American Dental Association. House Resolution 25-2006. The Community Dental Health Coordinator Proposal. ADA HOD 2006.

[74] American Dental Hygienists' Association. The Advanced Dental Hygiene Practitioner. Available at: http://www.adha.org/media/releases/archives/2004/070804_adhp.htm. Accessed September 1, 2007.

[75] Swider SM. Outcome effectiveness of community health workers: an integrative literature review. Public Health Nurs 2002;19(1):11–20.

[76] Reinschmidt KM, Hunter JB, Fernandez ML, et al. Understanding the success of promotoras in increasing chronic diseases screening. J Health Care Poor Underserved 2006;17(2): 256–64.

ELSEVIER
SAUNDERS

THE DENTAL
CLINICS
OF NORTH AMERICA

Dent Clin N Am 52 (2008) 463–467

Index

Note: Page numbers of article titles are in **boldface** type.